MW01470537

MEDITERRANEAN DASH DIET 2021

TASTY AND HEALTHY RECIPE BOOK FOR LOSING WEIGHT, REDUCING BLOOD PRESSURE AND DIABETES

Table of Contents

Introduction

The Mediterranean DASH diet is designed to help you lower your blood pressure, improve cardiac health, reduce the risk of cancer and type 2 diabetes, and, in some cases, lose weight. The Mediterranean diet is based on eating, cooking, and other lifestyle factors that focus on an abundance of whole foods. The DASH diet was created to avoid hypertension through the intake of some nutrients and others' elimination. These two diets overlap in many areas, but merging them fully creates a powerful duo that is sustainable—and delicious—for the long term. It's no wonder they've been the top two diets, as ranked by U.S. News & World Report, for many years running.

The combination of the two diets creates an exclusive method to the DASH diet that is extremely flexible, packed with vegetarian and pastry options, and it makes cooking at home or eating out easy and doable. Once you understand the basics and start building your recipe arsenal, customizing your favorite dishes will become second nature. You never have to be afraid of running out of recipe ideas!

As someone who has a deep love for both food and health, I've filled this book with satisfying dishes rooted in the flavorful culinary traditions of Greece, Italy, and Spain, among others, and included tips to make committing to this nutritionally balanced way of eating as easy as possible. I hope you'll find the information in this book and the recipes as useful and tasty as I do.

Enough of the pep talk. It's time to get started. Let's find out what the Mediterranean DASH diet is all about, how and why it was developed, and how you can use it to improve your health!

Chapter 1.   Breakfast and Smoothies Recipes

1. Mediterranean Pita Breakfast

Preparation Time: 22 minutes
Cooking Time: 3 minutes
Servings: 2
Difficulty Level: Easy
Ingredients:
- 1/4 cup of sweet red pepper
- 1/4 cup of chopped onion
- 1 cup of egg substitute
- 1/8 teaspoon of salt
- 1/8 teaspoon of pepper
- 1 small chopped tomato
- 1/2 cup of fresh torn baby spinach
- 1-1/2 teaspoons of minced fresh basil
- 2 whole size pita pieces of bread
- 2 tablespoons of crumbled feta cheese

Directions:

1. Coat with a cooking spray a small size non-stick skillet. Stir in the onion and red pepper for 3 minutes over medium heat. Add your egg substitute and season with salt and pepper. Stir cook until it sets.
2. Mix the torn spinach, chopped tomatoes, and mince basil. Scoop onto the pitas. Top vegetable mixture with your egg mixture.
3. Top with crumbled feta cheese and serve immediately.

Nutrition (for 100g):

- Calories: 267
- Fat: 3g
- Carbohydrates: 41g
- Protein: 20g
- Sodium: 643mg

2. Hummus Deviled Egg

Preparation Time: 10 minutes
Cooking Time: 0 minutes
Servings: 6
Difficulty Level: Easy
Ingredients:

- 1/4 cup of finely diced cucumber
- 1/4 cup of finely diced tomato
- 2 teaspoons of fresh lemon juice
- 1/8 teaspoon salt
- 6 hard-cooked peeled eggs, sliced half lengthwise
- 1/3 cup of roasted garlic hummus or any hummus flavor
- Chopped fresh parsley (optional)

Directions:

1. Combine the tomato, lemon juice, cucumber, and salt together, and then gently mix. Scrape out the yolks from the halved eggs and store them for later use.
2. Scoop a heaping teaspoon of hummus in each half egg.
3. Top with parsley and half-teaspoon tomato-cucumber mixture. Serve immediately.

Nutrition (for 100g):

- Calories: 40
- Fat: 1g
- Carbohydrates: 3g
- Protein: 4g
- Sodium: 544mg

3. Smoked Salmon Scrambled Egg

Preparation Time: 2 minutes
Cooking Time: 8 minutes
Servings: 4

Difficulty Level: Average
Ingredients:
- 16 ounces' egg substitute, cholesterol-free
- 1/8 teaspoon of black pepper
- 2 tablespoons of sliced green onions, keep the tops
- 1 ounce of chilled reduced-fat cream cheese, cut into 1/4-inch cubes
- 2 ounces of flaked smoked salmon

Directions:

1. Cut the chilled cream cheese into ¼-inch cubes, then set aside.
2. Whisk the egg substitute and the pepper in a large-sized bowl
3. Coat a non-stick skillet with cooking spray over medium heat. Stir in the egg substitute and cook for 5 to 7 minutes or until it starts to set, stirring occasionally and scraping the bottom of the pan.
4. Fold in the cream cheese, green onions, and salmon. Continue to cook and stir for another 3 minutes or just until the eggs are still moist but cooked.

Nutrition (for 100g):

- Calories: 100
- Fats: 3g
- Carbohydrates: 2g
- Protein: 15g
- Sodium: 772mg

4. Buckwheat Apple-Raisin Muffin

Preparation Time: 24 minutes
Cooking Time: 20 minutes
Servings: 12
Difficulty Level: Average
Ingredients:
- 1 cup of all-purpose flour
- 3/4 cup of buckwheat flour

- 2 tablespoons of brown sugar
- 1 1/2 teaspoons of baking powder
- 1/4 teaspoon of baking soda
- 3/4 cup of reduced-fat buttermilk
- 2 tablespoons of olive oil
- 1 large egg
- 1 cup peeled and cored, fresh diced apples
- 1/4 cup of golden raisins

Directions:

1. Prepare the oven at 375 ° F. Line a 12-cup muffin tin with a non-stick cooking spray or paper cups. Set aside. Incorporate all the dry ingredients in a mixing bowl. Set aside.
2. Beat together the liquid ingredients until smooth. Transfer the liquid mixture over the flour mixture and mix until moistened. Fold in the diced apples and raisins.
3. Fill each muffin cup with about 2/3 full of the mixture. Bake until it turns golden brown. Use the toothpick test. Serve.

Nutrition (for 100g):

- Calories: 117
- Fat: 1g
- Carbohydrates: 19g
- Protein: 3g
- Sodium: 683mg

5. Pumpkin Bran Muffin

Preparation Time: 20 minutes
Cooking Time: 20 minutes
Servings: 22
Difficulty Level: Average
Ingredients:

- 3/4 cup of all-purpose flour
- 3/4 cup of whole wheat flour
- 2 tablespoons sugar

- 1 tablespoon of baking powder
- 1/8 teaspoon salt
- 1 teaspoon of pumpkin pie spice
- 2 cups of 100% bran cereal
- 1 1/2 cups of skim milk
- 2 egg whites
- 15 ounces' x 1 can pumpkin
- 2 tablespoons of avocado oil

Directions:

1. Preheat the oven to 400 °F. Prepare a muffin pan enough for 22 muffins and line with a non-stick cooking spray. Stir together the first four ingredients until combined. Set aside.
2. Using a large mixing bowl, mix together milk and cereal bran and let it stand for 2 minutes or until the cereal softens. Add in the oil, egg whites, and pumpkin in the bran mix and blend well. Fill in the flour mixture and mix well.
3. Divide the batter into equal portions into the muffin pan. Bake for 20 minutes. Pull out the muffins from the pan and serve warm or cooled.

Nutrition (for 100g):

- Calories: 70
- Fat: 3g
- Carbohydrates: 14g
- Protein: 3g
- Sodium: 484mg

6. Buckwheat Buttermilk Pancakes

Preparation Time: 2 minutes
Cooking Time: 18 minutes
Servings: 9
Difficulty Level: Easy
Ingredients:
- 1/2 cup of buckwheat flour

- 1/2 cup of all-purpose flour
- 2 teaspoons of baking powder
- 1 teaspoon of brown sugar
- 2 tablespoons of olive oil
- 2 large eggs
- 1 cup of reduced-fat buttermilk

Directions:

1. Incorporate the first four ingredients in a bowl. Add the oil, buttermilk, and eggs and mix until thoroughly blended.
2. Put the griddle over medium heat and spray with non-stick cooking spray.
3. Pour ¼ cup of the batter over the skillet and cook for 1-2 minutes on each side or until they turn golden brown. Serve immediately.

Nutrition (for 100g):

- Calories: 108
- Fat: 3g
- Carbohydrates: 12g
- Protein: 4g
- Sodium: 556mg

7. French Toast with Almonds and Peach Compote

Preparation Time: 10 minutes
Cooking Time: 15 minutes
Servings: 4
Difficulty Level: Easy
Ingredients:
Compote:
- 3 tablespoons of sugar substitute, sucralose-based
- 1/3 cup + 2 tablespoons of water, divided
- 1 1/2 cups of fresh peeled or frozen, thawed and drained sliced peaches
- 2 tablespoons peach fruit spread, no-sugar-added

- 1/4 teaspoon of ground cinnamon

Almond French toast:

- 1/4 cup of (skim) fat-free milk
- 3 tablespoons of sugar substitute, sucralose-based
- 2 whole eggs
- 2 egg whites
- 1/2 teaspoon of almond extract
- 1/8 teaspoon salt
- 4 slices of multigrain bread
- 1/3 cup of sliced almonds

Directions:

1. To make the compote, dissolve 3 tablespoons sucralose in 1/3 cup of water in a medium saucepan over high-medium heat. Stir in the peaches and bring to a boil. Reduce the heat to medium and continue to cook uncovered for another 5 minutes or until the peaches softened.
2. Combine remaining water and fruit spread, then stir into the peaches in the saucepan. Cook for another minute or until syrup thickens. Pull out from heat and add in the cinnamon. Cover to keep warm.
3. To make the French toast. Combine the milk and sucralose in a large size shallow dish and whisk until it completely dissolves. Whisk in the egg whites, eggs, almond extract, and salt. Dip both sides of the bread slices for 3 minutes in the egg mixture or until completely soaked. Sprinkle both sides with sliced almonds and press firmly to adhere.
4. Brush the non-stick skillet with cooking spray and place over medium-high heat. Cook the bread slices on the griddle for 2 to 3 minutes on both sides or until it turns light brown. Serve topped with the peach compote.

Nutrition (for 100g):

- Calories: 277
- Fat: 7g
- Carbohydrates: 31g
- Protein: 12g; Sodium: 665mg

8. Mixed Berries Oatmeal with Sweet Vanilla Cream

Preparation Time: 5 minutes
Cooking Time: 5 minutes
Servings: 4
Difficulty Level: Easy
Ingredients:

- 2 cups of water
- 1 cup of quick-cooking oats
- 1 tablespoon of sucralose-based sugar substitute
- 1/2 teaspoon of ground cinnamon
- 1/8 teaspoon of salt

Cream:

- 3/4 cup of fat-free half-and-half
- 3 tablespoons of sucralose-based sugar substitute
- 1/2 teaspoon of vanilla extract
- 1/2 teaspoon of almond extract

Toppings:

- 1 1/2 cups of fresh blueberries
- 1/2 cup of fresh or frozen and thawed raspberries

Directions:

1. Boil water in high-heat and stir in the oats. Reduce heat to medium while cooking oats, uncovered for 2 minutes or until thick. Remove from heat and stir in sugar substitute, salt, and cinnamon.
2. In a medium-size bowl, incorporate all the cream ingredients until well blended. Scoop cooked oatmeal into 4 equal portions and pour the sweet cream over. Top with the berries and serve.

Nutrition (for 100g):

- Calories: 150
- Fat: 5g
- Carbohydrates: 30g
- Protein: 5g ; sodium: 807mg

9. Choco-Strawberry Crepe

Preparation Time: 5 minutes
Cooking Time: 10 minutes
Servings: 4
Difficulty Level: Easy
Ingredients:

- 1 cup of wheat all-purpose flour
- 2/3 cup of low-fat (1%) milk
- 2 egg whites
- 1 egg
- 3 tablespoons of sugar
- 3 tablespoons of unsweetened cocoa powder
- 1 tablespoon of cooled melted butter
- 1/2 teaspoon of salt
- 2 teaspoons of canola oil
- 3 tablespoons of strawberry fruit spread
- 3 1/2 cups of sliced thawed frozen or fresh strawberries
- 1/2 cup of fat-free thawed frozen whipped topping
- Fresh mint leaves (if desired)

Directions:

1. Incorporate the first eight ingredients in a large size bowl until smooth and thoroughly blended.
2. Brush ¼-teaspoon oil on a small size non-stick skillet over medium heat. Pour ¼-cup of the batter onto the center and swirl to coat the pan with batter.
3. Cook for a minute or until crêpe turns dull and the edges dry. Flip on the other side and cook for another half a minute. Repeat the process with the remaining mixture and oil.
4. Scoop ¼-cup of thawed strawberries at the center of the crepe and roll up to cover filling. Top with 2 tablespoons whipped cream and garnish with mint before serving.

Nutrition (for 100g):

- Calories: 334

- Fat: 5g
- Carbohydrates: 58g
- Protein: 10g
- Sodium: 678mg

10. No Crust Asparagus-Ham Quiche

Preparation Time: 5 minutes
Cooking Time: 42 minutes
Servings: 6
Difficulty Level: Easy
Ingredients:
- 2 cups 1/2-inched of sliced asparagus
- 1 red chopped bell pepper
- 1 cup of milk, low fat (1%)
- 2 tablespoons of wheat all-purpose flour
- 4 egg whites
- 1 egg, whole
- 1 cup of cooked chopped deli ham
- 2 tablespoons of fresh chopped tarragon or basil
- 1/2 teaspoon of salt (optional)
- 1/4 teaspoon of black pepper
- 1/2 cup of Swiss cheese, finely shredded

Directions:

1. Preheat your oven to 350 °F. Microwave bell pepper and asparagus in a tablespoon of water on HIGH for 2 minutes. Drain. Whisk flour and milk, and then add egg and egg whites until well combined. Stir in the vegetables and the remaining ingredients except for the cheese.
2. Pour in a 9-inch size pie dish and bake for 35 minutes. Sprinkle cheese over the quiche and bake another 5 minutes or until cheese melts. Allow it cool for 5 minutes, then cut into 6 wedges to serve.

Nutrition (for 100g):

- Calories 138
- Fat 1g
- Carbohydrates 8g
- Protein 13g
- Sodium 588mg

11. Apple Cheese Scones

Preparation Time: 20 minutes
Cooking Time: 15 minutes
Servings: 10
Difficulty Level: Average
Ingredients:
- 1 cup of all-purpose flour
- 1 cup of whole wheat flour, white
- 3 tablespoons of sugar
- 1 1/2 teaspoons of baking powder
- 1/2 teaspoon of salt
- 1/2 teaspoon of ground cinnamon
- 1/4 teaspoon of baking soda
- 1 diced Granny Smith apple
- 1/2 cup of shredded sharp Cheddar cheese
- 1/3 cup of applesauce, natural or unsweetened
- 1/4 cup of milk, fat-free (skim)
- 3 tablespoons of melted butter
- 1 egg

Directions:

1. Prepare your oven to 425 degrees F. Ready the baking sheet by lining it with parchment paper. Merge all dry ingredients in a bowl and mix. Stir in the cheese and apple. Set aside. Whisk all the wet ingredients together. Pour over the dry mixture until blended and turns like a sticky dough.

2. Work on the dough on a floured surface about 5 times. Pat and then stretch into an 8-inch circle. Slice into 10 diagonal cuts.
3. Place on the baking sheet and spray top with cooking spray. Bake for 15 minutes or until lightly golden. Serve.

Nutrition (for 100g):

- Calories 169
- Fat 2g
- Carbohydrates 26g
- Protein 5g
- Sodium 689mg

12. Bacon and Egg Wrap

Preparation Time: 15 minutes
Cooking Time: 15 minutes
Servings: 4
Difficulty Level: Easy
Ingredients:
- 1 cup of egg substitute, cholesterol-free
- 1/4 cup of Parmesan cheese, shredded
- 2 slices diced Canadian bacon
- 1/2 teaspoon of red hot pepper sauce
- 1/4 teaspoon of black pepper
- 4x7-inch whole wheat tortillas
- 1 cup of baby spinach leaves

Directions:

1. Preheat your oven at 325 ° F. Combine the first five ingredients to make the filling. Pour the mixture into a 9-inch glass dish sprayed with butter-flavored cooking spray.
2. Bake for 15 minutes or until the egg sets. Remove from oven. Place the tortillas for a minute in the oven. Cut baked egg mixture into quarters. Arrange one quarter at the center of each tortilla and top with ¼-cup spinach. Fold tortilla from the

bottom to the center and then both sides to the center to enclose. Serve immediately.

Nutrition (for 100g):

- Calories 195
- Fat 3g
- Carbohydrates 20g
- Protein 15g
- Sodium 688mg

13. Orange-Blueberry Muffin

Preparation Time: 10 minutes
Cooking Time: 10-25 minutes
Servings: 12
Difficulty Level: Average
Ingredients:
- 1 3/4 cups of all-purpose flour
- 1/3 cup of sugar
- 2 1/2 teaspoons of baking powder
- 1/2 teaspoon of baking soda
- 1/2 teaspoon of salt
- 1/2 teaspoon of ground cinnamon
- 3/4 cup of milk, fat-free (skim)
- 1/4 cup of butter
- 1 egg, large, lightly beaten
- 3 tablespoons of thawed orange juice concentrate
- 1 teaspoon of vanilla
- 3/4 cup of fresh blueberries

Directions:

1. Ready your oven to 400 ° F. Follow steps 2 to 5 of the Buckwheat Apple-Raisin Muffin recipe. Fill up the muffin cups ¾-full of the mixture and bake for 20 to 25 minutes. Let it cool for 5 minutes and serve warm.

Nutrition (for 100g):

- Calories 149
- Fat 5g
- Carbohydrates 24g
- Protein 3g
- Sodium 518mg

14. Baked Ginger Oatmeal with Pear Topping

Preparation Time: 10 minutes
Cooking Time: 15 minutes
Servings: 2
Difficulty Level: Easy
Ingredients:
- 1 cup of old-fashioned oats
- 3/4 cup of milk, fat-free (skim)
- 1 egg white
- 1 1/2 teaspoons of grated ginger, fresh or 3/4 teaspoon of ground ginger
- 2 tablespoons of brown sugar, divided
- 1/2 ripe diced pear

Directions:

1. Spray 2x6 ounce ramekins with a non-stick cooking spray. Prepare the oven to 350 ° F. Combine the first four ingredients and a tablespoon of sugar, then mix well. Pour evenly between the 2 ramekins. Top with pear slices and the remaining tablespoon of sugar. Bake for 15 minutes. Serve warm.

Nutrition (for 100g):

- Calories 268
- Fat 5g
- Carbohydrates 2g
- Protein 10g
- Sodium 779mg

15. Greek-Style Veggie Omelet

Preparation Time: 10 minutes
Cooking Time: 20 minutes
Servings: 2
Difficulty Level: Easy
Ingredients:

- 4 large eggs
- 2 tablespoons of fat-free milk
- 1/8 teaspoon of salt
- 3 teaspoons of olive oil, divided
- 2 cups of baby Portobello, sliced
- 1/4 cup of finely chopped onion
- 1 cup of fresh baby spinach
- 3 tablespoons of feta cheese, crumbled
- 2 tablespoons of ripe olives, sliced
- Freshly ground pepper

Directions:

1. Whisk together the first three ingredients. Stir in 2 tablespoons of oil in a non-stick skillet over medium-high heat. Sauté the onions and mushroom for 5-6 minutes or until golden brown. Mix in the spinach and cook. Remove mixture from pan.
2. Using the same pan, heat over medium-low heat the remaining oil. Pour your egg mixture and as it starts to set, pushed the edges towards the center to let the uncooked mixture flow underneath. When eggs are set, scoop the veggie mixture on one side. Sprinkle with olives and feta, then fold the other side to close. Slice in half and sprinkle with pepper to serve.

Nutrition (for 100g):

- Calories 271
- Fat 2g
- Carbohydrates 7g
- Protein 18g
- Sodium 648mg

16. Sweet Potatoes with Coconut Flakes

Preparation Time: 15 mins
Cooking Time: 1 hour
Servings: 2
Ingredients:

- 16 oz.. of sweet potatoes
- 1 tbsp. of maple syrup
- ¼ c. of Fat-free coconut Greek yogurt
- 1/8 c. of unsweetened toasted coconut flakes
- 1 chopped apple

Directions:

1. Preheat oven to 400 °F.
2. Place your potatoes on a baking sheet. Bake them for 45 - 60 minutes or until soft.
3. Use a sharp knife to mark "X" on the potatoes and fluff pulp with a fork.
4. Top with coconut flakes, chopped apple, Greek yogurt, and maple syrup.
5. Serve immediately.

Nutrition:

- Calories: 321; Fat: 3 g; Carbs: 70 g; Protein: 7 g; Sugars: 0.1 g; Sodium: 3%

17. Flaxseed & Banana Smoothie

Preparation Time: 5 mins
Cooking Time: 0 mins
Servings: 1
Ingredients:

- 1 frozen banana

- ½ c. of almond milk
- Vanilla extract.
- 1 tbsp. of almond butter
- 2 tbsps. of Flax seed 1 tsp. maple syrup

Directions:

1. Add all your ingredients to a food processor or blender and run until smooth. Pour the mixture into a glass and enjoy.

Nutrition:

- Calories: 376
- Fat: 19.4 g
- Carbs: 48.3 g
- Protein: 9.2 g
- Sugars: 12%
- Sodium: 64.9 mg

18. Fruity Tofu Smoothie

Preparation Time: 5 mins
Cooking Time: 0 mins
Servings: 2
Ingredients:

- 1 c. of ice cold water
- 1 c. of packed spinach
- ¼ c. of frozen mango chunks
- ½ c. of frozen pineapple chunks
- 1 tbsp. of chia seeds
- 1 container of silken tofu
- 1 frozen medium banana

Directions:

1. In a powerful blender, add all ingredients and puree until smooth and creamy.

2. Evenly divide into two glasses, serve and enjoy.

Nutrition:

- Calories: 175
- Fat: 3.7 g
- Carbs: 33.3 g
- Protein: 6.0 g
- Sugars: 16.3 g
- Sodium: 1%

19. French Toast with Applesauce

Preparation Time: 5 mins
Cooking Time: 5 mins
Servings: 6
Ingredients:

- ¼ c. of unsweetened applesauce
- ½ c. of skim milk
- 2 packets of Stevia
- 2 eggs
- 6 slices of whole-wheat bread
- 1 tsp. of ground cinnamon

Directions:

1. Mix well applesauce, sugar, cinnamon, milk, and eggs in a mixing bowl.
2. One slice at a time, soak the bread into an applesauce mixture until wet.
3. On medium fire, heat a large nonstick skillet.
4. Add soaked bread on one side and another on the other side. Cook in a single layer in batches for 2-3 minutes per side on medium-low fire or until lightly browned.
5. Serve and enjoy.

Nutrition:

- Calories: 122.6
- Fat: 2.6 g
- Carbs: 18.3 g
- Protein: 6.5 g
- Sugars: 14.8 g
- Sodium: 11%

20. Banana-Peanut Butter 'n Greens Smoothie

Preparation Time: 5 mins
Cooking Time: 0 mins
Servings: 1
Ingredients:

- 1 c. of chopped and packed Romaine lettuce
- 1 frozen medium banana
- 1 tbsp. of all-natural peanut butter
- 1 c. of cold almond milk

Directions:

1. In a heavy-duty blender, add all ingredients.
2. Puree until smooth and creamy.
3. Serve and enjoy.

Nutrition:

- Calories: 349.3
- Fat: 9.7 g
- Carbs: 57.4 g
- Protein: 8.1 g
- Sugars: 4.3 g
- Sodium: 18%

21. Baking Powder Biscuits

Preparation Time: 5 mins

Cooking Time: 5 mins
Servings: 1
Ingredients:

- 1 egg white
- 1 c. of white whole-wheat flour
- 4 tbsps. of Non-hydrogenated vegetable shortening
- 1 tbsp. of sugar
- 2/3 c. of low-fat milk
- 1 c. of unbleached all-purpose flour
- 4 tsps. of Sodium-free baking powder

Directions:

1. Preheat oven to 450°F. Take out a baking sheet and set it aside.
2. Place the flour, sugar, and baking powder into a mixing bowl and whisk well to combine.
3. Cut the shortening into the mixture using your fingers, and work until it resembles coarse crumbs. Add the egg white and milk and stir to combine.
4. Turn the dough out onto a lightly floured surface and knead for 1 minute. Roll dough to ¾ inch thickness and cut into 12 rounds.
5. Place rounds on the baking sheet. Place baking sheet on middle rack in the oven and bake 10 minutes.
6. Remove baking sheet and place biscuits on a wire rack to cool.

Nutrition:

- Calories: 118
- Fat: 4 g
- Carbs: 16 g
- Protein: 3 g
- Sugars: 0.2 g
- Sodium: 6%

22. Oatmeal Banana Pancakes with Walnuts

Preparation Time: 15 mins
Cooking Time: 5 mins
Servings: 8 pancakes
Ingredients:

- 1 finely diced firm banana
- 1 c. of whole wheat pancake mix
- 1/8 c. of chopped walnuts
- ¼ c. of old-fashioned oats

Directions:

1. Make the pancake mix according to the directions on the package.
2. Add walnuts, oats, and chopped banana.
3. Coat a griddle with cooking spray. Add about ¼ cup of the pancake batter onto the griddle when hot.
4. Turn pancake over when bubbles form on top. Cook until golden brown.
5. Serve immediately.

Nutrition:

- Calories: 155
- Fat: 4 g
- Carbs: 28 g
- Protein: 7 g
- Sugars: 2.2 g ; Sodium: 16%

23. Creamy Oats, Greens & Blueberry Smoothie

Preparation Time: 4 mins
Cooking Time: 0 mins
Servings: 1
Ingredients:

- 1 c. of cold Fat-free milk
- 1 c. of salad greens

- ½ c. of fresh frozen blueberries
- ½ c. of frozen cooked oatmeal
- 1 tbsp. of sunflower seeds

Directions:

1. In a powerful blender, blend all ingredients until smooth and creamy.
2. Serve and enjoy.

Nutrition:

- Calories: 280
- Fat: 6.8 g
- Carbs: 44.0 g
- Protein: 14.0 g
- Sugars: 32 g
- Sodium: 141%

24. Banana & Cinnamon Oatmeal

Preparation Time: 5 mins
Cooking Time: 0 mins
Servings: 6
Ingredients:

- 2 c. of quick-cooking oats
- 4 c. of Fat-free milk
- 1 tsp. of ground cinnamon
- 2 chopped large ripe banana
- 4 tsps. of Brown sugar
- Extra ground cinnamon

Directions:

1. Place milk in a skillet and bring to boil. Add oats and cook over medium heat until thickened, for two to four minutes. Stir intermittently.

2. Add cinnamon, brown sugar, banana, and stir to combine.
3. If you want, serve with the extra cinnamon and milk. Enjoy!

Nutrition:

- Calories: 215
- Fat: 2 g
- Carbs: 42 g
- Protein: 10 g
- Sugars: 1 g
- Sodium: 40%

25. Bagels Made Healthy

Preparation Time: 5 mins
Cooking Time: 40 mins
Servings: 8

Ingredients:

- 1 ½ c. of warm water
- 1 ¼ c. of bread flour
- 2 tbsps. of Honey
- 2 c. of whole wheat flour
- 2 tsps. of Yeast
- 1 ½ tbsps. of Olive oil
- 1 tbsp. of vinegar

Directions:

1. In a bread machine, mix all ingredients, and then process on dough cycle.
2. Once done, create 8 pieces shaped like a flattened ball.
3. Make a hole in the center of each ball using your thumb then create a donut shape.
4. In a greased baking sheet, place donut-shaped dough then covers and let it rise about ½ hour.

5. Prepare about 2 inches of water to boil in a large pan.
6. In a boiling water, drop one at a time the bagels and boil for 1 minute, then turn them once.
7. Remove them and return to a baking sheet and bake at 350oF for about 20 to 25 minutes until golden brown.

Nutrition:

- Calories: 228.1
- Fat: 3.7 g
- Carbs: 41.8 g
- Protein: 6.9 g
- Sugars: 0 g
- Sodium: 15%

Chapter 2.   Lunch Recipes

26. Rice with Vermicelli

Preparation Time: 5 minutes
Cooking Time: 45 minutes
Servings: 6
Difficulty Level: Easy
Ingredients:
- 2 cups of short-grain rice
- 3½ cups of water, plus more for rinsing and soaking the rice
- ¼ cup of olive oil
- 1 cup of broken vermicelli pasta
- Salt

Directions:

1. Soak the rice under cold water until the water runs clear. Place the rice in a bowl, cover with water, and let soak for 10 minutes. Drain and set aside. Cook the olive oil in a medium pot over medium heat.
2. Stir in the vermicelli and cook for 2 to 3 minutes, stirring continuously, until golden.
3. Put the rice and cook for 1 minute, stirring, so the rice is well coated in the oil. Stir in the water and a pinch of salt and bring the liquid to a boil. Adjust heat and simmer for 20 minutes. Pull out from the heat and let rest for 10 minutes. Fluff with a fork and serve.

Nutrition (for 100g):

- Calories 346
- Total fat 9g
- Carbohydrates 60g
- Protein 2g
- Sodium 0.9mg

27. Fava Beans and Rice

Preparation Time: 10 minutes
Cooking Time: 35 minutes
Servings: 4
Difficulty Level: Easy
Ingredients:

- ¼ cup of olive oil
- 4 cups of fresh fava beans, shelled
- 4½ cups of water, plus more for drizzling
- 2 cups of basmati rice
- 1/8 teaspoon of salt
- 1/8 teaspoon of freshly ground black pepper
- 2 tablespoons of pine nuts, toasted
- ½ cup of chopped fresh garlic chives or fresh onion chives

Directions:

1. Fill the saucepan with olive oil and cook over medium heat. Add the fava beans and drizzle them with a bit of water to avoid burning or sticking. Cook for 10 minutes.
2. Gently stir in the rice. Add the water, salt, and pepper. Set up the heat and boil the mixture. Adjust the heat and let it simmer for 15 minutes.
3. Pull out from the heat and let it rest for 10 minutes before serving. Spoon onto a serving platter and sprinkle with the toasted pine nuts and chives.

Nutrition (for 100g):

- Calories 587
- Total fat 17g
- Carbohydrates 97g
- Protein 2g
- Sodium 0.6mg

28. Buttered Fava Beans

Preparation Time: 30 minutes
Cooking Time: 15 minutes
Servings: 4
Difficulty Level: Easy
Ingredients:

- ½ cup of vegetable broth
- 4 pounds of fava beans, shelled
- ¼ cup of fresh tarragon, divided
- 1 teaspoon of chopped fresh thyme
- ¼ teaspoon of freshly ground black pepper
- 1/8 teaspoon of salt
- 2 tablespoons of butter
- 1 garlic clove, minced
- 2 tablespoons of chopped fresh parsley

Directions:

1. Boil the vegetable broth in a shallow pan over medium heat. Add the fava beans, 2 tablespoons of tarragon, thyme, pepper, and salt. Cook until the broth is almost absorbed and the beans are tender.
2. Stir in the butter, garlic, and remaining 2 tablespoons of tarragon. Cook for 2 to 3 minutes. Sprinkle with the parsley and serve hot.

Nutrition (for 100g):

- Calories 458
- Fat 9g
- Carbohydrates 81g
- Protein 37g
- Sodium 691mg

29. Freekeh

Preparation Time: 10 minutes
Cooking Time: 40 minutes
Servings: 4
Difficulty Level: Easy
Ingredients:

- 4 tablespoons of Ghee
- 1 onion, chopped
- 3½ cups of vegetable broth
- 1 teaspoon of ground allspice
- 2 cups of freekeh
- 2 tablespoons of pine nuts, toasted

Directions:

1. Melt ghee in a heavy-bottomed saucepan over medium heat. Stir in the onion and cook for about 5 minutes, constantly stirring, until the onion is golden.
2. Pour in the vegetable broth, add the allspice, and bring to a boil. Stir in the freekeh and return the mixture to a boil. Adjust heat and simmer for 30 minutes; stir occasionally.
3. Spoon the freekeh into a serving dish and top with the toasted pine nuts.

Nutrition (for 100g):

- Calories 459
- Fat 18g
- Carbohydrates 64g
- Protein 10g
- Sodium 692mg

30. Fried Rice Balls with Tomato Sauce

Preparation Time: 15 minutes
Cooking Time: 20 minutes
Servings: 8
Difficulty Level: Difficult
Ingredients:
- 1 cup of bread crumbs
- 2 cups of cooked risotto
- 2 large eggs, divided
- ¼ cup of freshly grated Parmesan cheese
- 8 fresh baby mozzarella balls, or 1 (4-inch) log fresh mozzarella, cut into 8 pieces
- 2 tablespoons of water
- 1 cup of corn oil
- 1 cup of Basic Tomato Basil Sauce, or store-bought

Directions:

1. Situate the breadcrumbs into a small bowl and set them aside. In a medium bowl, stir together the risotto, 1 egg, and the Parmesan cheese until well. Split the risotto mixture into 8 pieces. Situate them on a clean work surface and flatten each piece.
2. Place 1 mozzarella ball on each flattened rice disk. Close the rice around the mozzarella to form a ball. Repeat until you finish all the balls. In the same medium, now-empty bowl, whisk the remaining egg and the water. Dip each prepared risotto ball into the egg wash and roll it in the breadcrumbs. Set aside.
3. Cook corn oil in a skillet over high heat. Gently lower the risotto balls into the hot oil and fry for 5 to 8 minutes until golden brown. Stir them, as needed, to ensure the entire surface is fried. Using a slotted spoon, put the fried balls on paper towels to drain.
4. Warm up the tomato sauce in a medium saucepan over medium heat for 5 minutes, stir occasionally, and serve the warm sauce alongside the rice balls.

Nutrition (for 100g):

- Calories 255
- Fat 15g
- Carbohydrates 16g
- Protein 2g; Sodium 669mg

31. Spanish-Style Rice

Preparation Time: 10 minutes
Cooking Time: 35 minutes
Servings: 4
Difficulty Level: Average
Ingredients:

- ¼ cup olive oil
- 1 small onion, finely chopped
- 1 red bell pepper, seeded and diced
- 1½ cups white rice
- 1 teaspoon sweet paprika
- ½ teaspoon ground cumin
- ½ teaspoon ground coriander
- 1 garlic clove, minced
- 3 tablespoons tomato paste
- 3 cups vegetable broth
- 1/8 teaspoon salt

Directions:

1. Cook the olive oil in a large heavy-bottomed skillet over medium heat. Stir in the onion and red bell pepper. Cook for 5 minutes or until softened. Add the rice, paprika, cumin, and coriander and cook for 2 minutes, stirring often.
2. Add the garlic, tomato paste, vegetable broth, and salt. Stir it well and season, as needed. Allow the mixture to a boil. Lower heat and simmer for 20 minutes.
3. Set aside for 5 minutes before serving.

Nutrition (for 100g):

- Calories 414
- Fat 14g
- Carbohydrates 63g
- Protein 2g
- Sodium 664mg

32. Zucchini with Rice and Tzatziki

Preparation Time: 20 minutes
Cooking Time: 35 minutes
Servings: 4
Difficulty Level: Average
Ingredients:
- ¼ cup of olive oil
- 1 onion, chopped
- 3 zucchinis, diced
- 1 cup of vegetable broth
- ½ cup of chopped fresh dill
- Salt
- Freshly ground black pepper
- 1 cup of short-grain rice
- 2 tablespoons of pine nuts
- 1 cup of Tzatziki Sauce, Plain Yogurt, or store-bought

Directions:

1. Cook oil in a heavy-bottomed pot over medium heat. Stir in the onion, turn the heat to medium-low, and sauté for 5 minutes. Mix in the zucchini and cook for 2 minutes more.
2. Stir in the vegetable broth, dill, and season with salt and pepper. Turn up the heat to medium and bring the mixture to a boil.
3. Stir in the rice and place the mixture back to a boil. Set the heat to very low, cover the pot, and cook for 15 minutes. Pull out from the heat and set aside, for 10 minutes. Scoop the rice onto a serving platter, sprinkle with the pine nuts, and serve with tzatziki sauce.

Nutrition (for 100g):

- Calories 414
- Fat 17g
- Carbohydrates 57g
- Protein 5g
- Sodium 591mg

33. Cannellini Beans with Rosemary and Garlic Aioli

Preparation Time: 10 minutes
Cooking Time: 10 minutes
Servings: 4
Difficulty Level: Easy
Ingredients:
- 4 cups of cooked cannellini beans
- 4 cups of water
- ½ teaspoon of salt
- 3 tablespoons of olive oil
- 2 tablespoons of chopped fresh rosemary
- ½ cup of Garlic Aioli
- ¼ teaspoon of freshly ground black pepper

Directions:

1. Mix the cannellini beans, water, and salt in a medium saucepan over medium heat. Bring to a boil. Cook for 5 minutes. Drain. Cook the olive oil in a skillet over medium heat.
2. Add the beans. Stir in the rosemary and aioli. Adjust heat to medium-low and cook, stirring, just to heat through. Season with pepper and serve.

Nutrition (for 100g):

- Calories 545
- Fat 36g
- Carbohydrates 42g
- Protein 14g
- Sodium 608mg

34. Jeweled Rice

Preparation Time: 15 minutes
Cooking Time: 30 minutes
Servings: 6
Difficulty Level: Difficult
Ingredients:

- ½ cup of olive oil, divided
- 1 onion, finely chopped
- 1 garlic clove, minced
- ½ teaspoon of chopped peeled fresh ginger
- 4½ cups of water
- 1 teaspoon of salt, divided, plus more as needed
- 1 teaspoon of ground turmeric
- 2 cups of basmati rice
- 1 cup of fresh sweet peas
- 2 carrots, peeled and cut into ½-inch dice
- ½ cup of dried cranberries
- Grated zest of 1 orange
- 1/8 teaspoon of cayenne pepper
- ¼ cup of slivered almonds, toasted

Directions:

1. Warm up ¼ cup of olive oil in a large pan. Place the onion and cook for 4 minutes. Sauté in the garlic and ginger.
2. Stir in the water, ¾ teaspoon of salt, and turmeric. Bring the mixture to a boil. Put in the rice and return the mixture to a boil. Taste the broth and season with more salt, as needed. Select the heat to be low, and cook for 15 minutes. Turn off the heat. Let the rice rest on the burner, covered, for 10 minutes.
3. Meanwhile, in a medium sauté pan or skillet over medium-low heat, heat the remaining ¼ cup of olive oil. Stir in the peas and carrots. Cook for 5 minutes.
4. Stir in the cranberries and orange zest. Dust with the remaining salt and the cayenne. Cook for 1 to 2 minutes. Spoon the rice

onto a serving platter. Top with peas and carrots and sprinkle with toasted almonds.

Nutrition (for 100g):

- Calories 460
- Fat 19g
- Carbohydrates 65g
- Protein 4g
- Sodium 810mg

35. Asparagus Risotto

Preparation Time: 15 minutes
Cooking Time: 30 minutes
Servings: 4
Difficulty Level: Difficult
Ingredients:

- 5 cups of vegetable broth, divided
- 3 tablespoons of unsalted butter, divided
- 1 tablespoon of olive oil
- 1 small onion, chopped
- 1½ cups of Arborio rice
- 1-pound of fresh asparagus, ends trimmed, cut into 1-inch pieces, tips separated
- ¼ cup of freshly grated Parmesan cheese

Directions:

1. Boil the vegetable broth over medium heat. Set the heat to low and simmer. Mix 2 tablespoons of butter with olive oil. Stir in the onion and cook for 2 to 3 minutes.
2. Put the rice and stir with a wooden spoon while cooking for 1 minute until the grains are well covered with butter and oil.
3. Stir in ½ cup of warm broth. Cook and continue stirring until the broth is completely absorbed. Add the asparagus stalks and another ½-cup of broth. Cook and stir occasionally.

4. Continue adding the broth, ½ cup at a time, and cooking until it is completely absorbed upon adding the next ½-cup. Stir frequently to prevent sticking. Rice should be cooked but still firm.
5. Add the asparagus tips, the remaining 1-tablespoon of butter, and the Parmesan cheese. Stir vigorously to combine. Remove from the heat, top with additional Parmesan cheese, if desired, and serve immediately.

Nutrition (for 100g):

- Calories 434
- Fat 14g
- Carbohydrates 67g
- Protein 6g
- Sodium 517mg

36. Vegetable Paella

Preparation Time: 25 minutes
Cooking Time: 45 minutes
Servings: 6
Difficulty Level: Average
Ingredients:
- ¼ cup of olive oil
- 1 large sweet onion
- 1 large red bell pepper
- 1 large green bell pepper
- 3 garlic cloves, finely minced
- 1 teaspoon of smoked paprika
- 5 saffron threads
- 1 zucchini, cut into ½-inch cubes
- 4 large ripe tomatoes, peeled, seeded, and chopped
- 1½ cups of short-grain Spanish rice
- 3 cups of vegetable broth, warmed

Directions:

1. Preheat the oven to 350 °F. Cook the olive oil over medium heat. Stir in the onion and red and green bell peppers and cook for 10 minutes.
2. Stir in the garlic, paprika, saffron threads, zucchini, and tomatoes. Turn down the heat to medium-low and cook for 10 minutes.
3. Stir in the rice and vegetable broth. Increase the heat to bring the paella to a boil. Put the heat to medium-low and cook for 15 minutes. Wrap the pan with aluminum foil and put it in the oven.
4. Bake for 10 minutes or until the broth is absorbed.

Nutrition (for 100g):

- Calories 288
- Fat 10g
- Carbohydrates 46g
- Protein 3g
- Sodium 671mg

37. Eggplant and Rice Casserole

Preparation Time: 30 minutes
Cooking Time: 35 minutes
Servings: 4
Difficulty Level: Difficult
Ingredients:
For the Sauce:

- ½ cup of olive oil
- 1 small onion, chopped
- 4 garlic cloves, mashed
- 6 ripe tomatoes, peeled and chopped
- 2 tablespoons of tomato paste
- 1 teaspoon of dried oregano
- ¼ teaspoon of ground nutmeg
- ¼ teaspoon of ground cumin

For the Casserole:

- 4 (6-inch) Japanese eggplants, halved lengthwise
- 2 tablespoons of olive oil
- 1 cup of cooked rice
- 2 tablespoons of pine nuts, toasted
- 1 cup of water

Directions:
To Make the Sauce:

1. Cook the olive oil in a heavy-bottomed saucepan over medium heat. Place the onion and cook for 5 minutes. Stir in the garlic, tomatoes, tomato paste, oregano, nutmeg, and cumin. Bring to a boil, then reduce heat and simmer for 10 minutes. Remove and set aside.

To Make the Casserole:

1. Preheat the broiler. While the sauce simmers, drizzle the eggplant with the olive oil and place them on a baking sheet. Broil for about 5 minutes until golden. Remove and let cool. Turn the oven to 375 °F. Arrange the cooled eggplant, cut-side up, in a 9-by-13-inch baking dish. Gently scoop out some flesh to make room for the stuffing.
2. In a bowl, combine half the tomato sauce, the cooked rice, and pine nuts. Fill each eggplant half with the rice mixture. In the same bowl, combine the remaining tomato sauce and water. Pour over the eggplant. Bake, covered, for 20 minutes until the eggplant is soft.

Nutrition (for 100g):

- Calories 453
- Fat 39g
- Carbohydrates29g
- Protein7g
- Sodium 820mg

38. Many Vegetable Couscous

Preparation Time: 15 minutes
Cooking Time: 45 minutes
Servings: 8
Difficulty Level: Difficult
Ingredients:

- ¼ cup of olive oil
- 1 onion, chopped
- 4 garlic cloves, minced
- 2 jalapeño peppers, pierced with a fork in several places
- ½ teaspoon of ground cumin
- ½ teaspoon of ground coriander
- 1 (28-ounce) can of crushed tomatoes
- 2 tablespoons of tomato paste
- 1/8 teaspoon of salt
- 2 bay leaves
- 11 cups of water, divided
- 4 carrots
- 2 zucchinis, cut into 2-inch pieces
- 1 acorn squash, halved, seeded, and cut into 1-inch-thick slices
- 1 (15-ounce) can of chickpeas, drained and rinsed
- ¼ cup of chopped Preserved Lemons (optional)
- 3 cups of couscous

Directions:

1. Cook the olive oil in a heavy-bottom pot. Place the onion and cook for 4 minutes. Stir in the garlic, jalapeños, cumin, and coriander. Cook for 1 minute. Add the tomatoes, tomato paste, salt, bay leaves, and 8 cups of water. Bring the mixture to a boil.
2. Add the carrots, zucchini, and acorn squash and return to a boil. Reduce the heat slightly, cover, and cook for about 20 minutes until the vegetables are tender but not mushy. Get 2 cups of the cooking liquid and set aside. Season as needed.
3. Add the chickpeas and preserved lemons (if using). Cook for few minutes, and turn off the heat.

4. In a medium pan, bring the remaining 3 cups of water to a boil over high heat. Stir in the couscous, cover, and turn off the heat. Let the couscous rest for 10 minutes. Drizzle with 1 cup of the reserved cooking liquid. Using a fork, fluff the couscous.
5. Mound it on a large platter. Drizzle it with the remaining cooking liquid. Pull out the vegetables from the pot and arrange them on top. Serve the remaining stew in a separate bowl.

Nutrition (for 100g):

- Calories 415
- Fat 7g
- Carbohydrates 75g
- Protein 9g
- Sodium 718mg

39. Kushari

Preparation Time: 25 minutes
Cooking Time: 1 hour and 20 minutes
Servings: 8
Difficulty Level: Difficult
Ingredients:
For the sauce:
- 2 tablespoons of olive oil
- 2 garlic cloves, minced
- 1 (16-ounce) can of tomato sauce
- ¼ cup of white vinegar
- ¼ cup of Harissa, or store-bought
- 1/8 teaspoon of salt

For the rice:
- 1 cup of olive oil
- 2 onions, thinly sliced
- 2 cups of dried brown lentils
- 4 quarts plus ½ cup of water, divided

- 2 cups of short-grain rice
- 1 teaspoon of salt
- 1-pound of short elbow pasta
- 1 (15-ounce) can of chickpeas, drained and rinsed

Directions:
To make the sauce:

1. In a saucepan, cook the olive oil. Sauté the garlic. Stir in the tomato sauce, vinegar, harissa, and salt. Bring the sauce to a boil. Turn down the heat to low and cook for 20 minutes or until the sauce has thickened. Remove and set aside.

To make the rice

1. Ready the plate with paper towels and set aside. In a large pan over medium heat, heat the olive oil. Sauté the onions, often stir, until crisp and golden. Transfer the onions to the prepared plate and set them aside. Reserve 2 tablespoons of the cooking oil. Reserve the pan.
2. Over high heat, combine the lentils and 4 cups of water in a pot. Allow it to boil and cook for 20 minutes. Strain and toss with the reserved 2 tablespoons of cooking oil. Set aside. Reserve the pot.
3. Place the pan you used to fry the onions over medium-high heat and add the rice, 4½ cups of water, and salt. Bring to a boil. Set the heat to low, and cook for 20 minutes. Turn off and set aside for 10 minutes. Bring the remaining 8 cups of water, salted, to a boil over high heat in the same pot used to cook the lentils. Drop in the pasta and cook for 6 minutes or according to the package instructions. Drain and set aside.

To assemble:

1. Spoon the rice onto a serving platter. Top it with lentils, chickpeas, and pasta. Drizzle with the hot tomato sauce and sprinkle with the crispy fried onions.

Nutrition (for 100g):

- Calories668
- Fat 13g
- Carbohydrates 113g
- Protein 18g
- Sodium 481mg

40. Bulgur with Tomatoes and Chickpeas

Preparation Time: 10 minutes
Cooking Time: 35 minutes
Servings: 6
Difficulty Level: Average
Ingredients:

- ½ cup of olive oil
- 1 onion, chopped
- 6 tomatoes, diced, or 1 (16-ounce) can diced tomatoes
- 2 tablespoons of tomato paste
- 2 cups of water
- 1 tablespoon of Harissa, or store-bought
- 1/8 teaspoon of salt
- 2 cups of coarse bulgur
- 1 (15-ounce) can of chickpeas, drained and rinsed

Directions:

1. In a heavy-bottomed pot over medium heat, heat the olive oil. Sauté the onion, then add the tomatoes with their juice and cook for 5 minutes.
2. Stir in the tomato paste, water, harissa, and salt. Bring to a boil.
3. Stir in the bulgur and chickpeas. Return the mixture to a boil. Decrease the heat to low and cook for 15 minutes. Let rest for 15 minutes before serving.

Nutrition (for 100g):

- Calories 413
- Fat 19g
- Carbohydrates 55g
- Protein 14g
- Sodium 728mg

41. Mackerel Maccheroni

Preparation Time: 10 minutes
Cooking Time: 15 minutes
Servings: 4
Difficulty Level: Easy
Ingredients:

- 12 oz. of Maccheroni
- 1 clove garlic
- 14 oz. of Tomato sauce
- 1 sprig chopped parsley
- 2 Fresh chili peppers
- 1 teaspoon of salt
- 7 oz. of mackerel in oil
- 3 tablespoons of extra virgin olive oil

Directions:

1. Start by putting the water to a boil in a saucepan. While the water is heating up, take a pan, pour in a little oil and a little garlic, and cook over low heat. Once the garlic is cooked, pull it out from the pan.
2. Cut open the chili pepper, remove the internal seeds and cut into thin strips.
3. Add the cooking water and the chili pepper to the same pan as before. Then, take the mackerel, and after draining the oil and separating it with a fork, put it in the pan with the other ingredients. Lightly sauté it by adding some cooking water.
4. When all the ingredients are well incorporated, add the tomato puree to the pan. Mix well to even out all the ingredients and cook on low heat for about 3 minutes.

Let's move on to the pasta:

1. After the water starts boiling, add the salt and the pasta. Drain the maccheroni once they are slightly al dente, and add them to the sauce you prepared.
2. Sauté for a few moments in the sauce and after tasting, season with salt and pepper according to your liking.

Nutrition (for 100g):

- Calories 510
- Fat 15.4g
- Carbohydrates 70g
- Protein 22.9g
- Sodium 730mg

42. Maccheroni with Cherry Tomatoes and Anchovies

Preparation Time: 10 minutes
Cooking Time: 15 minutes
Servings: 4
Difficulty Level: Easy
Ingredients:
- 14 oz. of Maccheroni Pasta
- 6 Salted anchovies
- 4 oz. of Cherry tomatoes
- 1 clove garlic
- 3 tablespoons of extra virgin olive oil
- Fresh chili peppers to taste
- 3 basil leaves
- Salt to taste

Directions:

1. Start by heating water in a pot and add salt when it is boiling. Meanwhile, prepare the sauce: take the tomatoes after having washed them and cut them into 4 pieces.

2. Now, take a non-stick pan, sprinkle in a little oil, and throw in a clove of garlic. Once cooked, remove it from the pan. Add the clean anchovies to the pan, melting them in the oil.
3. When the anchovies are well dissolved, add the cut tomatoes pieces and turn the heat up to high until they begin to soften (be careful not to let them become too soft).
4. Add the chili peppers without seeds, cut into small pieces, and season.
5. Transfer the pasta to the pot of boiling water, drain it al dente, and let it sauté in the saucepan for a few moments.

Nutrition (for 100g):

- Calories 476
- Fat 11g
- Carbohydrates 81.4g
- Protein 12.9g
- Sodium 763mg

43. Lemon and Shrimp Risotto

Preparation Time: 10 minutes
Cooking Time: 30 minutes
Servings: 4
Difficulty Level: Easy
Ingredients:
- 1 lemon
- 14 oz. of Shelled shrimp
- 1 ¾ cups of risotto rice
- 1 white onion
- 33 fl. oz. (1 liter) of vegetable broth (even less is fine)
- 2 ½ tablespoons of butter
- ½ glass of white wine
- Salt to taste
- Black pepper to taste
- Chives to taste

Directions:

1. Start by boiling the shrimps in salted water for 3-4 minutes, drain and set aside.
2. Peel and finely chop an onion, stir-fry it with melted butter and once the butter has dried, toast the rice in the pan for a few minutes.
3. Deglaze the rice with half a glass of white wine, then add the juice of 1 lemon. Stir and finish cooking the rice by continuing to add a spoon of vegetable stock as needed.
4. Mix well and a few minutes before the end of cooking, add the previously cooked shrimps (keeping some of them aside for garnish) and some black pepper.
5. Once the heat is off, add a knob of butter and stir. The risotto is ready to be served. Decorate with the remaining shrimp and sprinkle with some chives.

Nutrition (for 100g):

- Calories 510
- Fat 10g
- Carbohydrates 82.4g
- Protein 20.6g
44. Sodium 875mg

44. Spaghetti with Clams

Preparation Time: 10 minutes
Cooking Time: 40 minutes
Servings: 4
Difficulty Level: Easy
Ingredients:
- 11.5 oz. of spaghetti
- 2 pounds of clams
- 7 oz. of tomato sauce, or tomato pulp, for the red version of this dish
- 2 cloves of garlic

- 4 tablespoons of extra virgin olive oil
- 1 glass of dry white wine
- 1 tablespoon of finely chopped parsley
- 1 chili pepper

Directions:

1. Start by washing the clams: never "purge" the clams—they must only be opened through the use of heat; otherwise, their precious internal liquid is lost along with any sand. Wash the clams quickly using a colander placed in a salad bowl: this will filter out the sand on the shells.
2. Then immediately put the drained clams in a saucepan with a lid on high heat. Turn them over occasionally, and when they are almost all open, take them off the heat. The clams that remain closed are dead and must be eliminated. Remove the mollusks from the open ones, leaving some of them whole to decorate the dishes. Strain the liquid left at the bottom of the pan, and set it aside.
3. Take a large pan and pour a little oil into it. Heat a whole pepper and one or two cloves of crushed garlic on very low heat until the cloves become yellowish. Add the clams and season with dry white wine.
4. Now, add the clam liquid strained previously and some finely chopped parsley.
5. Strain and immediately toss the spaghetti al dente in the pan after having cooked them in plenty of salted water. Stir well until the spaghetti absorbs all the liquid from the clams. If you did not use a chili pepper, complete with a light sprinkle of white or black pepper.

Nutrition (for 100g):

- Calories 167
- Fat 8g
- Carbohydrates 8.63g
- Protein 5g
- Sodium 720mg

45. Greek Fish Soup

Preparation Time: 10 minutes
Cooking Time: 60 minutes
Servings: 4
Difficulty Level: Easy
Ingredients:
- Hake or other white fish
- 4 Potatoes
- 4 Spring onions
- 2 Carrots
- 2 stalks of Celery
- 2 Tomatoes
- 4 tablespoons of Extra virgin olive oil
- 2 Eggs
- 1 Lemon
- 1 cup of Rice
- Salt to taste

Directions:

1. Choose a fish not exceeding 2.2pounds in weight, remove its scales, gills, and intestines and wash it well. Salt it and set it aside.
2. Wash the potatoes, carrots, and onions and put them in the saucepan whole with enough water to soak them and then bring to a boil.
3. Add in the celery still tied in bunches, so it does not disperse while cooking; cut the tomatoes into four parts and add these too, together with oil and salt.
4. When the vegetables are almost cooked, add more water and the fish. Boil for 20 minutes, then remove it from the broth together with the vegetables.
5. Place the fish in a serving dish by adorning it with the vegetables and strain the broth. Put the broth back on the heat, diluting it with a little water. Once it boils, put in the rice and season with salt. Once the rice is cooked, remove the saucepan from the heat.

Prepare the avgolemono sauce:

1. Beat the eggs well and slowly add the lemon juice. Put some broth in a ladle and slowly pour it into the eggs, mixing constantly.
2. Finally, add the obtained sauce to the soup and mix well.

Nutrition (for 100g):

- Calories 263
- Fat 17.1g
- Carbohydrates 18.6g
- Protein 9g
- Sodium 823mg

46. Venere Rice with Shrimp

Preparation Time: 10 minutes
Cooking Time: 55 minutes
Servings: 3
Difficulty Level: Easy
Ingredients:
- 1 ½ cups of black Venere rice (better if parboiled)
- 5 teaspoons of extra virgin olive oil
- 10.5 oz. of shrimp
- 10.5 oz. of zucchini
- 1 Lemon (juice and rind)
- Table Salt to taste
- Black pepper to taste
- 1 clove garlic
- Tabasco to taste

Directions:
Let's start with the rice:

1. After filling a pot with plenty of water and bringing it to a boil, pour in the rice, add salt, and cook for the necessary time (check the package's cooking instructions).

2. Meanwhile, grate the zucchini with a grater with large holes. In a pan, heat the olive oil with the peeled garlic clove, add the grated zucchini, salt, and pepper, cook for 5 minutes; remove the garlic clove, and set the vegetables aside.

Now clean the shrimp:

1. Remove the shell, cut the tail, divide them in half lengthwise, and remove the intestine (the dark thread in their back). Situate the cleaned shrimps in a bowl and season with olive oil; give it some extra flavor by adding lemon zest, salt, and pepper and by adding a few drops of Tabasco if you so choose.
2. Heat up the shrimps in a hot pan for a couple of minutes. Once cooked, set aside.
3. Once the Venere rice is ready, strain it in a bowl, add the zucchini mix, and stir.

Nutrition (for 100g):

- Calories 293
- Fat 5g
- Carbohydrates 52g
- Protein 10g
- Sodium 655mg

47. Pennette with Salmon and Vodka

Preparation Time: 10 minutes
Cooking Time: 18 minutes
Servings: 4
Difficulty Level: Easy
Ingredients:
- 14 oz. of Pennette Rigate
- 7 oz. of Smoked salmon
- 1.2 oz. of Shallot
- 1.35 fl. oz..(40ml) of Vodka
- 5 oz.. of cherry tomatoes

- 7 oz.. of fresh liquid cream (I recommend the vegetable one for a lighter dish)
- Chives to taste
- 3 tablespoons of extra virgin olive oil
- Salt to taste
- Black pepper to taste
- Basil to taste (for garnish)

Directions:

1. Wash and cut the tomatoes and the chives. After having peeled the shallot, chop it with a knife, put it in a saucepan, and let it marinate in extra virgin olive oil for a few moments.
2. Meanwhile, cut the salmon into strips and sauté it together with the oil and shallot.
3. Blend everything with the vodka, being careful as there could be a flare (if a flame should rise, don't worry, it will lower as soon as the alcohol has evaporated completely). Add the chopped tomatoes and add a pinch of salt and, if you like, some pepper. Finally, add the cream and chopped chives.
4. While the sauce continues cooking, prepare the pasta. Once the water boils, pour in the Pennette and let them cook until al dente.
5. Strain the pasta, and pour the Pennette into the sauce, letting them cook for a few moments so as allow them to absorb all the flavor. If you like, garnish with a basil leaf.

Nutrition (for 100g):

- Calories 620
- Fat 21.9g
- Carbohydrates81.7g
- Protein 24g
- Sodium 326mg

48. Seafood Carbonara

Preparation Time: 15 minutes
Cooking Time: 50 minutes
Servings: 3

Difficulty Level: Easy
Ingredients:

- 11.5 oz. of Spaghetti
- 3.5 oz. of Tuna
- 3.5 oz. of Swordfish
- 3.5 oz. of Salmon
- 6 Yolks
- 4 tablespoons of Parmesan cheese (Parmigiano Reggiano)
- 2 fl. oz.. (60ml) of White wine
- 1 clove garlic
- Extra virgin olive oil to taste
- Table Salt to taste
- Black pepper to taste

Directions:

1. Prepare a boiling water in a pot and add a little salt.
2. Meanwhile, pour 6 egg yolks in a bowl and add the grated parmesan, pepper, and salt. Beat with a whisk, and dilute with a little cooking water from the pot.
3. Remove any bones from the salmon, the scales from the swordfish, and proceed by dicing the tuna, salmon, and swordfish.
4. Once it boils, toss in the pasta and cook it slightly al dente.
5. Meanwhile, heat a little oil in a large pan, add the whole peeled garlic clove. Once the oil is hot, toss in the fish cubes and sauté over high heat for about 1 minute. Remove the garlic and add the white wine.
6. Once the alcohol evaporates, take out the fish cubes and lower the heat. As soon as the spaghetti is ready, add them to the pan and sauté for about a minute, stirring constantly and adding the cooking water, as needed.
7. Pour in the egg yolk mixture and the fish cubes. Mix well. Serve.

Nutrition (for 100g):

- Calories 375
- Fat 17g
- Carbohydrates 41.40g

- Protein 14g
- Sodium 755 mg

49. Garganelli with Zucchini Pesto and Shrimp

Preparation Time: 10 minutes
Cooking Time: 30 minutes
Servings: 4
Difficulty Level: Average
Ingredients:
- 14 oz. egg-based Garganelli
- For the zucchini pesto:
- 7oz. Zucchini
- 1 cup Pine nuts
- 8 tablespoons (0.35oz.) Basil
- 1 teaspoon of table salt
- 9 tablespoons extra virgin olive oil
- 2 tablespoons Parmesan cheese to be grated
- 1oz. of Pecorino to be grated
- For the sautéed shrimp:
- 8.8oz. shrimp
- 1 clove garlic
- 7 teaspoons extra virgin olive oil
- Pinch of Salt

Directions:
Start by preparing the pesto:

1. After washing the zucchini, grate them, place them in a colander (to allow them to lose some excess liquid), and lightly salt them. Put the pine nuts, zucchini and basil leaves in the blender. Add the grated Parmesan, the pecorino, and the extra virgin olive oil.
2. Blend everything until the mixture is creamy, stir in a pinch of salt, and set aside.

Switch to the shrimp:

1. First of all, pull out the intestine by cutting the shrimp's back with a knife along its entire length and, with the tip of the knife, remove the black thread inside.
2. Cook the clove of garlic in a non-stick pan with extra virgin olive oil. When it's browned, remove the garlic and add the shrimps. Sauté them for about 5 minutes over medium heat until you see a crispy crust form on the outside.
3. Then, boil a pot of salted water and cook the Garganelli. Set a couple of spoons of cooking water aside, and drain the pasta al dente.
4. Put the Garganelli in the pan where you cooked the shrimp. Cook together for a minute, add a spoon of cooking water and finally, add the zucchini pesto.
5. Mix everything well to combine the pasta with the sauce.

Nutrition (for 100g):

*   Calories 776
*   Fat 46g
*   Carbohydrates 68g
*   Protein 22.5g
*   Sodium 835mg

50. Salmon Risotto

Preparation Time: 10 minutes
Cooking Time: 30 minutes
Servings: 4
Difficulty Level: Average
Ingredients:
*   1 ¾ cup (12.3 oz..) of Rice
*   8.8 oz. of Salmon steaks
*   1 Leek
*   Extra virgin olive oil to taste
*   1 clove of garlic

- ½ glass of white wine
- 3 ½ tablespoons of grated Grana Padano
- salt to taste
- Black pepper to taste
- 17 fl. oz. (500ml) of Fish broth
- 1 cup of butter

Directions:

1. Start by cleaning the salmon and cutting it into small pieces. Cook 1 tablespoon of oil in a pan with a whole garlic clove and brown the salmon for 2/3 minutes, add salt, and set the salmon aside, removing the garlic.

Now, start preparing the risotto:

1. Cut the leek into very small pieces and let it simmer in a pan over low heat with two oil tablespoons. Stir in the rice and cook it for a few seconds over medium-high heat, stirring with a wooden spoon.
2. Stir in the white wine, continue cooking, stir occasionally, try not to let the rice stick to the pan, and gradually add the stock (vegetable or fish).
3. Halfway through cooking, add the salmon, butter, and a pinch of salt if necessary. When the rice is well cooked, remove it from heat. Combine with a couple of tablespoons of grated Grana Padano and serve.

Nutrition (for 100g):

- Calories 521
- Fat 13g
- Carbohydrates 82g
- Protein 19g
- Sodium 839mg

Chapter 3.   Dinner Recipes

51. Spinach Rolls

Preparation Time: 10 minutes
Cooking Time: 10 minutes
Servings: 4
Ingredients:

- 4 eggs, whisked
- 1/3 cup of organic almond milk
- ½ teaspoon of salt
- ½ teaspoon of white pepper
- 1 teaspoon of butter
- 9 oz.. of chicken breast, boneless, skinless, cooked
- 2 cups of spinach
- 2 tablespoons of heavy cream

Directions:

1. Mix up together whisked eggs with almond milk and salt.
2. Preheat the skillet well and toss the butter in it.
3. Melt it.
4. Cook 4 crepes in the preheated skillet.
5. Meanwhile, chop the spinach and chicken breast.
6. Fill every egg crepe with chopped spinach, chicken breast, and heavy cream.
7. Roll the crepes and transfer them to the serving plate.

Nutrition:

- Calories 220
- Fat 14.5
- Fiber 0.8
- Carbs 2.4
- Protein 20.1
- Sodium 31%

52. Goat Cheese Fold-Overs

Preparation Time: 15 minutes
Cooking Time: 8 minutes
Servings: 4
Ingredients:

- 8 oz.. of goat cheese, crumbled
- 5 oz.. of ham, sliced
- 1 cup of almond flour
- ¼ cup of coconut milk
- 1 teaspoon of olive oil
- ½ teaspoon of dried dill
- 1 teaspoon of Italian seasoning
- ½ teaspoon of salt

Directions:

1. In the mixing bowl, mix up together almond flour, coconut milk, olive oil, and salt. You will get a smooth batter.
2. Preheat the non-stick skillet.
3. Separate batter into 4 parts. Pour 1st batter part in the preheated skillet and cook it for 1 minute from each side.
4. Repeat the same steps with all batter.
5. After this, mix up together crumbled goat cheese, dried dill, and Italian seasoning.
6. Spread every almond flour pancake with the goat cheese mixture. Add sliced ham and fold them.

Nutrition:

- Calories 402
- Fat 31.8
- Fiber 1.6
- Carbs 5.1
- Protein 25.1; Sodium 69%

53. Crepe Pie

Preparation Time: 10 minutes
Cooking Time: 15 minutes
Servings: 8
Ingredients:

- 1 cup of almond flour
- 1 cup of coconut flour
- ½ cup of heavy cream
- 1 teaspoon of baking powder
- ½ teaspoon of salt
- 10 oz.. of ham, sliced
- ½ cup of cream cheese
- 1 teaspoon of chili flakes
- 1 tablespoon of fresh cilantro, chopped
- 4 oz.. of Cheddar cheese, shredded

Directions:

1. Make crepes: in the mixing bowl, mix up together almond flour, coconut flour, heavy cream, salt, and baking powder. Whisk the mixture.
2. Preheat the non-stick skillet well and ladle 1 ladle of the crepe batter in it.
3. Make the crepes: cook them for 1 minute from each side over medium heat.
4. Mix up together cream cheese, chili flakes, cilantro, and shredded Cheddar cheese.
5. After this, transfer 1st crepe to the plate. Spread it with the cream cheese mixture. Add ham.
6. Repeat the steps until you use all the ingredients.
7. Bake the crepe pie for 5 minutes in the preheated to 365 °F oven.
8. Cut it into the serving and serve hot.

Nutrition:

- Calories 272
- Fat 18.8
- Fiber 6.9
- Carbs 13.2
- Protein 13.4
- Sodium 59%

54. Coconut Soup

Preparation Time: 15 minutes
Cooking Time: 25 minutes
Servings: 4
Ingredients:

- 1 cup of coconut milk
- 2 cups of water 1 teaspoon curry paste
- 4 chicken thighs
- ½ teaspoon of fresh ginger, grated
- 1 garlic clove, diced 1 teaspoon butter
- 1 teaspoon of chili flakes
- 1 tablespoon of lemon juice

Directions:

1. Toss the butter in the skillet and melt it.
2. Add diced garlic and grated ginger. Cook the ingredients for 1 minute. Stir them constantly.
3. Pour water into the saucepan. Add coconut milk and curry paste. Mix up the liquid until homogenous.
4. Add chicken thighs, chili flakes, and cooked ginger mixture. Close the lid and cook soup for 15 minutes.
5. Then start to whisk soup with the hand whisker and add lemon juice.
6. When all lemon juice is added, stop whisking it. Close the lid and cook soup for 5 minutes more over medium heat.
7. Then remove soup from the heat and let it rest for 15 minutes.

Nutrition:

- Calories 318
- Fat 26
- Fiber 1.4
- Carbs 4.2
- Protein 20.6
- Sodium 14%

55. Fish Tacos

Preparation Time: 10 minutes
Cooking Time: 5 minutes
Servings: 4
Ingredients:

- 4 lettuce leaves
- ½ red onion, diced
- ½ jalapeno pepper, minced
- 1 tablespoon of olive oil
- 1-pound of cod fillet
- 1 tablespoon of lemon juice
- ¼ teaspoon of ground coriander

Directions:

1. Sprinkle cod fillet with a ½ tablespoon of olive oil and ground coriander.
2. Preheat the grill well.
3. Grill the fish for 2 minutes from each side. The cooked fish has a light brown color.
4. After this, mix up together diced red onion, minced jalapeno pepper, remaining olive oil, and lemon juice.
5. Cut the grilled cod fillet into 4 pieces.
6. Place the fish in the lettuce leaves. Add a mixed red onion mixture over the fish and transfer the tacos to the serving plates.

Nutrition:

- Calories 157
- Fat 4.5
- Fiber 0.4
- Carbs 1.6
- Protein 26.1
- Sodium 37%

56. Cobb Salad

Preparation Time: 10 minutes
Cooking Time: 5 minutes
Servings: 2
Ingredients:

- 2 oz. of bacon, sliced
- 1 egg boiled, peeled
- ½ tomato, chopped
- 1 oz. of Blue cheese
- 1 teaspoon of chives
- 1/3 cup of lettuce, chopped
- 1 tablespoon of mayonnaise
- 1 tablespoon of lemon juice

Directions:

1. Place the bacon in the preheated skillet and roast it 1.5 minutes from each side.
2. When the bacon is cooked, chop it roughly and transfer it to the salad bowl.
3. Chop the eggs roughly and add them to the salad bowl too.
4. After this, add chopped tomato, chives, and lettuce.
5. Chop Blue cheese and add it to the salad.
6. Then make seasoning: whisk together mayonnaise with lemon juice.
7. Pour the mixture over the salad and shake a little.

Nutrition:

- Calories 270
- Fat 20.7
- Fiber 0.3
- Carbs 3.7
- Protein 16.6
- Sodium 43%

57. Cheese Soup

Preparation Time: 10 minutes
Cooking Time: 15 minutes
Servings: 3
Ingredients:

- 2 white onions, peeled, diced
- 1 cup of Cheddar cheese, shredded
- ½ cup of heavy cream
- ½ cup of water
- 1 teaspoon of ground black pepper
- 1 tablespoon of butter
- ½ teaspoon of salt

Directions:

1. Pour water and heavy cream into the saucepan.
2. Bring it to a boil.
3. Meanwhile, toss the butter in the pan, add diced onions and sauté them.
4. When the onions are translucent, transfer them to the boiling liquid.
5. Add ground black pepper, salt, and cheese. Cook the soup for 5 minutes.
6. Then let it chill little and ladle it into the bowls.

Nutrition:

- Calories 286
- Fat 23.8
- Fiber 1.8
- Carbs 8.3
- Protein 10.7
- Sodium 29%

58. Tuna Tartare

Preparation Time: 10 minutes
Cooking Time: 0 minutes
Servings: 4
Ingredients:

- 1-pound of tuna steak
- 1 tablespoon of mayonnaise
- 3 oz.. of avocado, chopped
- 1 cucumber, chopped
- 1 tablespoon of lemon juice
- 1 teaspoon of cayenne pepper
- 1 teaspoon of soy sauce
- 1 teaspoon of chives
- ½ teaspoon of cumin seeds
- 1 teaspoon of canola oil

Directions:

1. Chop tuna steak and place it in the big bowl.
2. Add avocado, cucumber, and chives.
3. Mix up together lemon juice, cayenne pepper, soy sauce, cumin seeds, canola oil, and mayonnaise.
4. Add mixed liquid in the tuna mixture and mix up well.
5. Place tuna tartare on the serving plates.

Nutrition:

- Calories 292
- Fat 13.9
- Fiber 2
- Carbs 6
- Protein 35.1
- Sodium 22%

59. Clam Chowder

Preparation Time: 5 minutes
Cooking Time: 15 minutes
Servings: 3
Ingredients:

- 1 cup of coconut milk
- 1 cup of water 6 oz.. clam, chopped
- 1 teaspoon of chives ½ teaspoon white pepper
- ¾ teaspoon of chili flakes ½ teaspoon salt
- 1 cup of broccoli florets, chopped

Directions:

1. Pour coconut milk and water into the saucepan.
2. Add chopped clams, chives, white pepper, chili flakes, salt, and broccoli florets.
3. Close the lid and cook chowder over medium-low heat for 15 minutes or until all the ingredients are soft.
4. It is recommended to serve the soup hot.

Nutrition:

- Calories 139
- Fat 9.8
- Fiber 1.1
- Carbs 10.8

- Protein 2.4
- Sodium 44%

60. Asian Beef Salad

Preparation Time: 10 minutes
Cooking Time: 25 minutes
Servings: 4
Ingredients:

- 14 oz.. of beef brisket
- 1 teaspoon of sesame seeds
- ½ teaspoon of cumin seeds
- 1 tablespoon of apple cider vinegar
- 1 tablespoon of avocado oil
- 1 red bell pepper, sliced
- 1 white onion, sliced
- 1 teaspoon of butter
- 1 teaspoon of ground black pepper
- 1 teaspoon of soy sauce
- 1 garlic clove, sliced
- 1 cup of water for cooking

Directions:

1. Slice beef brisket and place it in the pan. Add water and close the lid.
2. Cook the beef for 25 minutes.
3. Then drain water and transfer beef brisket to the pan.
4. Add butter and roast it for 5 minutes.
5. Put the cooked beef brisket in the salad bowl.
6. Add sesame seeds, cumin seeds, apple cider vinegar, avocado oil, sliced bell pepper, onion, ground black pepper, and soy sauce.
7. Sprinkle the salad with garlic and mix it up.

Nutrition:

- Calories 227
- Fat 8.1
- Fiber 1.4
- Carbs 6
- Protein 31.1
- Sodium 83%

61. Carbonara

Preparation Time: 10 minutes
Cooking Time: 25 minutes
Servings: 6
Ingredients:

- 3 zucchinis, trimmed
- 1 cup of heavy cream
- 5 oz.. of bacon, chopped
- 2 egg yolks
- 4 oz.. of Cheddar cheese, grated
- 1 tablespoon of butter
- 1 teaspoon of chili flakes
- 1 teaspoon of salt
- ½ cup of water, for cooking

Directions:

1. Make the zucchini noodles with the help of the spiralizer.
2. Toss bacon in the skillet and roast it for 5 minutes on medium heat. Stir it from time to time.
3. Meanwhile, in the saucepan, mix up together heavy cream, butter, salt, and chili flakes.
4. Add egg yolk and whisk the mixture until smooth.
5. Start to preheat the liquid, stir it constantly.
6. When the liquid starts to boil, add grated cheese and fried bacon. Mix it up and close the lid. Sauté it on the low heat for 5 minutes.
7. Meanwhile, place the zucchini noodles in the skillet where bacon was and roast it for 3 minutes.

8. Then pour heavy cream mixture over zucchini and mix up well. Cook it for 1 minute more and transfer it to the serving plates.

Nutrition:

- Calories 324
- Fat 27.1
- Fiber 1.1
- Carbs 4.6
- Protein 16
- Sodium 65%

62. Cauliflower Soup with Seeds

Preparation Time: 10 minutes
Cooking Time: 20 minutes
Servings: 4
Ingredients:

- 2 cups of cauliflower
- 1 tablespoon of pumpkin seeds
- 1 tablespoon of chia seeds
- ½ teaspoon of salt
- 1 teaspoon of butter
- ¼ white onion, diced
- ½ cup of coconut cream
- 1 cup of water
- 4 oz.. of Parmesan, grated
- 1 teaspoon of paprika
- 1 tablespoon of dried cilantro

Directions:

1. Chop cauliflower and put it in the saucepan.
2. Add salt, butter, diced onion, paprika, and dried cilantro.
3. Cook the cauliflower over medium heat for 5 minutes.

4. Then add coconut cream and water.
5. Close the lid and boil soup for 15 minutes.
6. Then blend the soup with the help of a hand blender.
7. Bring to boil it again.
8. Add grated cheese and mix up well.
9. Ladle the soup into the serving bowls and top every bowl with pumpkin seeds and chia seeds.

Nutrition:

- Calories 214
- Fat 16.4
- Fiber 3.6
- Carbs 8.1
- Protein 12.1
- Sodium 43%

63. Prosciutto-Wrapped Asparagus

Preparation Time: 15 minutes
Cooking Time: 20 minutes
Servings: 6
Ingredients:

- 2-pound of asparagus
- 8 oz.. of prosciutto, sliced
- 1 tablespoon of butter, melted
- ½ teaspoon of ground black pepper
- 4 tablespoons of heavy cream
- 1 tablespoon of lemon juice

Directions:

1. Slice prosciutto slices into strips.
2. Wrap asparagus into prosciutto strips and place on the tray.
3. Sprinkle the vegetables with ground black pepper, heavy cream, and lemon juice. Add butter.
4. Preheat the oven to 365 °F.

5. Place the tray with asparagus in the oven and cook for 20 minutes.
6. Serve the cooked meal only hot.

Nutrition:

- Calories 138
- Fat 7.9
- Fiber 3.2
- Carbs 6.9
- Protein 11.5
- Sodium 3%

64. Stuffed Bell Peppers

Preparation Time: 10 minutes
Cooking Time: 25 minutes
Servings: 4
Ingredients:

- 4 bell peppers
- 1 ½ cup of ground beef 1 zucchini, grated
- 1 white onion, diced
- ½ teaspoon of ground nutmeg
- 1 tablespoon of olive oil
- 1 teaspoon of ground black pepper
- ½ teaspoon of salt
- 3 oz. Parmesan, grated

Directions:

1. Cut the bell peppers into halves and remove seeds.
2. Place ground beef in the skillet.
3. Add grated zucchini, diced onion, ground nutmeg, olive oil, ground black pepper, and salt.
4. Roast the mixture for 5 minutes.
5. Place bell pepper halves in the tray.

6. Fill every pepper half with ground beef mixture and top with grated Parmesan.
7. Cover the tray with foil and secure the edges.
8. Cook the stuffed bell peppers for 20 minutes at 360°F.

Nutrition:

- Calories 241
- Fat 14.6
- Fiber 3.4
- Carbs 11
- Protein 18.6
- Sodium 37%

65. Stuffed Eggplants with Goat Cheese

Preparation Time: 15 minutes
Cooking Time: 25 minutes
Servings: 4
Ingredients:

- 1 large eggplant, trimmed
- 1 tomato, crushed
- 1 garlic clove, diced
- ½ teaspoon of ground black pepper
- ½ teaspoon of smoked paprika
- 1 cup of spinach, chopped
- 4 oz.. of goat cheese, crumbled
- 1 teaspoon of butter
- 2 oz.. of Cheddar cheese, shredded

Directions:

1. Cut the eggplants into halves and then cut every half into 2 parts.
2. Remove the flesh from the eggplants to get eggplant boards.

3. Mix up together crushed tomato, diced garlic, ground black pepper, smoked paprika, chopped spinach, crumbled goat cheese, and butter.
4. Fill the eggplants with this mixture.
5. Top every eggplant board with shredded Cheddar cheese.
6. Put the eggplants in the tray.
7. Preheat the oven to 365 °F.
8. Place the tray with eggplants in the oven and cook for 25 minutes.

Nutrition:

- Calories 229
- Fat 16.1
- Fiber 4.6
- Carbs 9
- Protein 13.8
- Sodium 21%

66. Korma Curry

Preparation Time: 10 minutes
Cooking Time: 25 minutes
Servings: 6
Ingredients:

- 3-pound of chicken breast, skinless, boneless
- 1 teaspoon of garam masala
- 1 teaspoon of curry powder
- 1 tablespoon of apple cider vinegar
- ½ teaspoon of coconut cream
- 1 cup of organic almond milk
- 1 teaspoon of ground coriander
- ¾ teaspoon of ground cardamom
- ½ teaspoon of ginger powder
- ¼ teaspoon of cayenne pepper
- ¾ teaspoon of ground cinnamon

- 1 tomato, diced 1 teaspoon avocado oil
- ½ cup of water

Directions:

1. Chop the chicken breast and put it in the saucepan.
2. Add avocado oil and start to cook it over medium heat.
3. Sprinkle the chicken with garam masala, curry powder, apple cider vinegar, ground coriander, cardamom, ginger powder, cayenne pepper, ground cinnamon, and diced tomato. Mix up the ingredients carefully. Cook them for 10 minutes.
4. Add water, coconut cream, and almond milk. Sauté the meat for 10 minutes more.

Nutrition:

- Calories 411
- Fat 19.3
- Fiber 0.9
- Carbs 6
- Protein 49.9
- Sodium 12%

67. Zucchini Bars

Preparation Time: 10 minutes
Cooking Time: 15 minutes
Servings: 8
Ingredients:

- 3 zucchinis, grated
- ½ white onion, diced
- 2 teaspoons of butter
- 3 eggs, whisked
- 4 tablespoons of coconut flour
- 1 teaspoon of salt
- ½ teaspoon of ground black pepper

- 5 oz.. of goat cheese, crumbled
- ½ cup of spinach, chopped
- 1 teaspoon of baking powder
- ½ teaspoon of lemon juice

Directions:

1. In the mixing bowl, mix up together grated zucchini, diced onion, eggs, coconut flour, salt, ground black pepper, crumbled cheese, chopped spinach, baking powder, and lemon juice.
2. Add butter and churn the mixture until homogenous.
3. Line the baking dish with baking paper.
4. Transfer the zucchini mixture to the baking dish and flatten it.
5. Preheat the oven to 365°F and put the dish inside.
6. Cook it for 15 minutes. Then chill the meal well.
7. Cut it into bars.

Nutrition:

- Calories 199
- Fat 1316
- Fiber 215
- Carbs 7.1
- Protein 13.1
- Sodium 21%

68. Mushroom Soup

Preparation Time: 10 minutes
Cooking Time: 25 minutes
Servings: 4
Ingredients:

- 1 cup of water
- 1 cup of coconut milk
- 1 cup of white mushrooms, chopped
- ½ carrot, chopped

- ¼ white onion, diced
- 1 tablespoon of butter
- 2 oz.. of turnip, chopped
- 1 teaspoon of dried dill
- ½ teaspoon of ground black pepper
- ¾ teaspoon of smoked paprika
- 1 oz.. of celery stalk, chopped

Directions:

1. Pour water and coconut milk into the saucepan. Bring the liquid to a boil. Add chopped mushrooms, carrots, and turnips. Close the lid and boil for 10 minutes.
2. Meanwhile, put butter in the skillet. Add diced onion. Sprinkle it with dill, ground black pepper, and smoked paprika. Roast the onion for 3 minutes. Add the roasted onion to the soup mixture.
3. Then add chopped celery stalk. Close the lid.
4. Cook soup for 10 minutes.
5. Then ladle it into the serving bowls.

Nutrition:

- Calories 181
- Fat 17.3
- Fiber 2.5
- Carbs 6.9
- Protein 2.4; Sodium 4%

69. Stuffed Portobello Mushrooms

Preparation Time: 10 minutes
Cooking Time: 10 minutes
Servings: 4
Ingredients:

- 2 Portobello mushrooms
- 2 oz.. of artichoke hearts, drained, chopped

- 1 tablespoon of coconut cream
- 1 tablespoon of cream cheese
- 1 teaspoon of minced garlic
- 1 tablespoon of fresh cilantro, chopped
- 3 oz.. of Cheddar cheese, grated
- ½ teaspoon of ground black pepper
- 2 tablespoons of olive oil
- ½ teaspoon of salt

Directions:

1. Sprinkle mushrooms with olive oil and place them in the tray. Transfer the tray in the preheated oven to 360 °F and broil them for 5 minutes.
2. Meanwhile, blend together artichoke hearts, coconut cream, cream cheese, minced garlic, and chopped cilantro. Add grated cheese in the mixture and sprinkle with ground black pepper and salt. Fill the broiled mushrooms with the cheese mixture and cook them for 5 minutes more. Serve the mushrooms only hot.

Nutrition:

- Calories 183
- Fat 16.3
- Fiber 1.9
- Carbs 3
- Protein 7.7; Sodium 37%

70. Lettuce Salad

Preparation Time: 10 minutes
Cooking Time: 0 minutes
Servings: 1
Ingredients:

- 1 cup of Romaine lettuce, roughly chopped
- 3 oz. of seitan, chopped

- 1 tablespoon of avocado oil
- 1 teaspoon of sunflower seeds
- 1 teaspoon of lemon juice
- 1 egg boiled, peeled
- 2 oz. of Cheddar cheese, shredded

Directions:

1. Place lettuce in the salad bowl. Add chopped seitan and Cheddar cheese.
2. Then chop the egg roughly and add it to the salad bowl too.
3. Mix up together lemon juice with the avocado oil.
4. Sprinkle the salad with the oil mixture and sunflower seeds. Don't stir the salad before serving.

Nutrition:

- Calories 663
- Fat 29.5
- Fiber 4.7
- Carbs 3.8
- Protein 84.2
- Sodium 45%

71. Lemon Garlic Salmon

Preparation Time: 3 minutes
Cooking Time: 17 minutes
Servings: 4
Ingredients:

- 2 pounds of salmon fillets, frozen
- 1 cup of water
- ¼ teaspoon of garlic powder
- 1/8 teaspoon of pepper
- ¼ cup of lemon juice
- ¼ teaspoon of salt to taste
- 1 lemon

Directions:

1. Put water into the instant pot and the lemon juice, then add the herbs and put it in a steamer rack.
2. Drizzle salmon with oil and season with pepper and salt.
3. Add garlic powder over salmon.
4. Layer the lemon slices over salmon.
5. Cook on manual high pressure for 7 minutes, then natural pressure release.
6. Enjoy over salad or some roasted veggies!

Nutrition:

- Calories: 165
- Fat: 10gg
- Carbs: 8g
- Net Carbs: 4g
- Protein: 15g
- Fiber: 4g
- Sodium 75%

72. Chickpea Curry

Preparation Time: 10 minutes
Cooking Time: 10 minutes
Servings: 6
Ingredients:

- 2 tablespoons of olive oil
- 1 diced small green pepper
- 2 cans of chickpeas, drained
- 1 cup of corn
- 1 cup of kale leaves
- 1 tablespoon of sugar-free maple syrup
- 1 diced onion
- 2 minced cloves of garlic
- 1 can of diced tomatoes with juice

- 1 cup of sliced okra
- 1 cup of vegetable broth
- 1 teaspoon of sea salt
- Juice of a lime
- ¼ teaspoon of ground black pepper
- 2 tablespoons of cilantro leaves

Directions:

1. Turn on the sauté function on the instant pot.
2. Cook onion for four minutes until browned, and then add in garlic and pepper and cook for 2 more minutes.
3. Add in curry powder and stir for 30 seconds, and then add the rest of the ingredients and seal the vent.
4. Cook under manual pressure for 5 minutes and then release natural pressure.
5. Add in the salt, pepper, and lime juice, and add more salt as needed.
6. Serve over cooked rice or top with cilantro leaves.

Nutrition:

- Calories: 119
- Fat: 5g
- Carbs: 18g
- Net Carbs: 16g
- Protein: 2g
- Fiber: 2g
- Sodium 30%

73. Instant Pot Chicken Thighs with Olives and Capers

Preparation Time: 15 minutes
Cooking Time: 20 minutes
Servings: 6
Ingredients:

- 6 chicken thighs
- 3 tablespoons of avocado oil
- ¼ teaspoon of sweet paprika
- A couple of small lemons
- 1 cup of chicken stock
- 1 cup of pitted olives
- 3 tablespoons of parsley leaves for garnish
- 1 teaspoon of kosher salt
- 1 teaspoon of ground turmeric
- ¼ teaspoon of black pepper
- ¼ teaspoon of mustard powder
- 2 tablespoons of cooking fat of choice
- 2 chopped cloves of garlic
- 2 tablespoons of capers

Directions:

1. Season chicken thighs with salt and put them in a baking dish.
2. Mix the spices with the avocado oil, put it over the chicken, put the marinate in there, and marinate for 20-30 minutes.
3. Halve the lemons, and then heat the ghee, swirling to the pot bottom. Brown the chickens for 3 minutes undisturbed, and then brown the second side.
4. Do this with the rest of the chicken, and then use the broth to deglaze the pot.
5. Put lemons at the bottom and chicken over the top, and then the rest of the ingredients over the chicken.
6. Let it cook for 14 minutes.
7. When finished, let natural pressure release, and then taste to see if it's ready, and put olives and capers over the chicken, garnishing with parsley.

Nutrition:

- Calories: 253
- Fat: 6g
- Carbs: 10gNet
- Carbs: 6g

- Protein: 13g
- Fiber: 4g
- Sodium 60%

74. Instant Pot salmon

Preparation Time: 5 minutes
Cooking Time: 15 minutes
Servings: 4
Ingredients:

- 1 cup of water
- 1 pound of salmon, cut into fillets
- Salt and pepper to taste

Directions:

1. Put a cup of water into the instant pot and add the trivet.
2. Put the fillets on top of that and add the salt and pepper onto it.
3. Secure and turn on the release valve to seal, and then cook on manual high pressure for 3 minutes or 5 minutes for frozen fillets.
4. When finished, let it vent and release the pressure, and serve with sauce or side dish.

Nutrition:

- Calories: 161
- Fat: 4g
- Carbs: 0
- Net Carbs: 0
- Protein: 22g
- Fiber: 0g
- Sodium 33%

75. Instant Pot Mac N' Cheese

Preparation Time: 10 minutes
Cooking Time: 10 minutes
Servings: 6
Ingredients:

- 1 cup of raw cashews, soaked
- ¼ cup of Nutritional yeast
- 1 tablespoon of apple cider vinegar
- 12 ounces of gluten-free pasta
- 5 cups of water, divided
- 2 teaspoons of sea salt
- 2 tablespoons of lemon juice
- 1//4 teaspoon of nutmeg

Directions:

1. Drain cashews and then combine them with 2 cups of water, yeast, lemon juice, vinegar, and nutmeg, and then blend until smooth.
2. Add pasta to the instant pot, put sauce on top, use two cups of water to rinse out the blender, pour water from the blender into the instant pot, and then seal and cook on manual pressure for 0 minutes, then let it natural pressure release.
3. Release steam and then put the rest of the water into a pot and use a spoon to stir.
4. Adjust seasonings, and you can add veggies and such to this.

Nutrition:

- Calories: 329
- Fat: 10g
- Carbs: 52g
- Net Carbs: 50g
- Protein: 7g ; Fiber: 2g ; Sodium 84%

Chapter 4.   Poultry and Meat Recipes

76. Mediterranean Pork Roast

Preparation Time: 10 minutes
Cooking Time: 8 hours and 10 minutes
Servings: 6
Difficulty Level: Average
Ingredients:

- 2 tablespoons of Olive oil
- 2 pounds of Pork roast
- ½ teaspoon of Paprika
- ¾ cup of Chicken broth
- 2 teaspoons of Dried Sage
- ½ tablespoon of Garlic minced
- ¼ teaspoon of Dried marjoram
- ¼ teaspoon of Dried Rosemary
- 1 teaspoon of Oregano
- ¼ teaspoon of Dried thyme
- 1 teaspoon of Basil
- ¼ teaspoon of Kosher salt

Directions:

1. In a small bowl, mix broth, oil, salt, and spices. In a skillet, pour olive oil and bring to medium-high heat. Put the pork into it and roast until all sides become brown.
2. Take out the pork after cooking and poke the roast all over with a knife. Place the poked pork roast into a 6-quart crockpot. Now, pour the small bowl mixture liquid all over the roast.
3. Seal crockpot and cook on low for 8 hours. After cooking, remove it from the crockpot onto a cutting board and shred it into pieces. Afterward, add the shredded pork back into the

crockpot. Simmer it another 10 minutes. Serve along with feta cheese, pita bread, and tomatoes.

Nutrition (for 100g):

- Calories 361
- Fat 10.4g
- Carbohydrates 0.7g
- Protein 43.8g
- Sodium 980mg

77. Beef Pizza

Preparation Time: 20 minutes
Cooking Time: 50 minutes
Servings: 10
Difficulty Level: Difficult
Ingredients:
For Crust:

- 3 cups of all-purpose flour
- 1 tablespoon of sugar
- 2¼ teaspoons of active dry yeast
- 1 teaspoon of salt
- 2 tablespoons of olive oil
- 1 cup of warm water

For Topping:

- 1-pound of ground beef
- 1 medium onion, chopped
- 2 tablespoons of tomato paste
- 1 tablespoon of ground cumin
- Salt and ground black pepper, as required
- ¼ cup of water
- 1 cup of fresh spinach, chopped
- 8 ounces of artichoke hearts, quartered
- 4 ounces of fresh mushrooms, sliced
- 2 tomatoes, chopped

- 4 ounces of feta cheese, crumbled

Directions:

For crust:

1. Mix the flour, sugar, yeast, and salt with a stand mixer, using the dough hook. Add 2 tablespoons of the oil and warm water and knead until a smooth and elastic dough is formed.
2. Make a ball of the dough and set it aside for about 15 minutes.
3. Situate the dough onto a lightly floured surface and roll into a circle. Situate the dough into a lightly, greased round pizza pan and gently press to fit. Set aside for about 10-15 minutes. Coat the crust with some oil. Preheat the oven to 400 ° F.

For topping:

1. Fry beef in a nonstick skillet over medium-high heat for about 4-5 minutes. Mix in the onion and cook for about 5 minutes, stirring frequently. Add the tomato paste, cumin, salt, black pepper, and water and stir to combine.
2. Set the heat to medium and cook for about 5-10 minutes. Remove from the heat and set aside. Place the beef mixture over the pizza crust and top with the spinach, followed by the artichokes, mushrooms, tomatoes, and Feta cheese.
3. Bake until the cheese is melted. Remove from the oven and set aside for about 3-5 minutes before slicing. Cut into desired-sized slices and serve.

Nutrition (for 100g):

- Calories 309
- Fat 8.7g
- Carbohydrates 3.7g
- Protein 3.3g
- Sodium 732mg

78. Beef & Bulgur Meatballs

Preparation Time: 20 minutes
Cooking Time: 28 minutes
Servings: 6
Difficulty Level: Average
Ingredients:

- ¾ cup of uncooked bulgur
- 1-pound of ground beef
- ¼ cup of shallots, minced
- ¼ cup of fresh parsley, minced
- ½ teaspoon of ground allspice
- ½ teaspoon of ground cumin
- ½ teaspoon of ground cinnamon
- ¼ teaspoon of red pepper flakes, crushed
- Salt, as required
- 1 tablespoon of olive oil

Directions:

1. In a large bowl with cold water, soak the bulgur for about 30 minutes. Drain the bulgur well, and then squeeze with your hands to remove the excess water. In a food processor, add the bulgur, beef, shallot, parsley, spices, salt, and pulse until a smooth mixture is formed.
2. Situate the mixture into a bowl and refrigerate, covered for about 30 minutes. Remove from the refrigerator and make equal-sized balls from the beef mixture. In a large nonstick skillet, heat the oil over medium-high heat and cook the meatballs in 2 batches for about 13-14 minutes, flipping frequently. Serve warm.

Nutrition (for 100g):

- Calories 228
- Fat7.4g
- Carbohydrates 0.1g
- Protein 3.5g
- Sodium 766mg

79. Tasty Beef and Broccoli

Preparation Time: 10 minutes
Cooking Time: 15 minutes
Servings: 4
Difficulty Level: Easy
Ingredients:

- 1 and ½ lbs. of flanks steak
- 1 tbsp. of olive oil
- 1 tbsp. of tamari sauce
- 1 cup of beef stock
- 1-pound of broccoli, florets separated

Directions:

1. Combine steak strips with oil and tamari, toss and set aside for 10 minutes. Select your instant pot on sauté mode, place beef strips, and brown them for 4 minutes on each side. Stir in stock, cover the pot again and cook on high for 8 minutes. Stir in broccoli, cover, and cook on high for 4 minutes more. Portion everything between plates and serve. Enjoy!

Nutrition (for 100g):

- Calories 312
- Fat 5g
- Carbohydrates 20g
- Protein 4g
- Sodium 694mg

80. Beef Corn Chili

Preparation Time: 8-10 minutes
Cooking Time: 30 minutes
Servings: 8
Difficulty Level: Average

Ingredients:

- 2 small onions, chopped (finely)
- ¼ cup of canned corn
- 1 tablespoon of oil
- 10 ounces of lean ground beef
- 2 small chili peppers, diced

Directions:

1. Turn on the instant pot. Click "SAUTE." Pour the oil, then stir in the onions, chili pepper, and beef; cook until turn translucent and softened. Pour the 3 cups water into the cooking pot; mix well.
2. Seal the lid and select "MEAT/STEW." Adjust the timer to 20 minutes. Allow to cook until the timer turns to zero.
3. Click "CANCEL" then "NPR" for natural release pressure for about 8-10 minutes. Open, and then place the dish on serving plates. Serve.

Nutrition (for 100g):

- Calories 94
- Fat 5g
- Carbohydrates 2g
- Protein 7g
- Sodium 477mg

81. Balsamic Beef Dish

Preparation Time: 5 minutes
Cooking Time: 55 minutes
Servings: 8
Difficulty Level: Average
Ingredients:
- 3 pounds of chuck roast
- 3 cloves garlic, thinly sliced
- 1 tablespoon of oil
- 1 teaspoon of flavored vinegar
- ½ teaspoon of pepper

- ½ teaspoon of rosemary
- 1 tablespoon of butter
- ½ teaspoon of thyme
- ¼ cup of balsamic vinegar
- 1 cup of beef broth

Directions:

1. Slice the slits in the roast and stuff in garlic slices all over. Combine flavored vinegar, rosemary, pepper, thyme and rub the mixture over the roast. Select the pot on sauté mode and mix in oil; allow the oil to heat up. Cook both sides of the roast.
2. Take it out and set it aside. Stir in butter, broth, balsamic vinegar, and deglaze the pot. Return the roast and close the lid, then cook on HIGH pressure for 40 minutes.
3. Perform a quick release. Serve!

Nutrition (for 100g):

- Calories 393
- Fat 15g
- Carbohydrates 25g
- Protein 37g
- Sodium 870mg

82. Soy Sauce Beef Roast

Preparation Time: 8 minutes
Cooking Time: 35 minutes
Servings: 2-3
Difficulty Level: Average
Ingredients:
- ½ teaspoon of beef bouillon
- 1 ½ teaspoon of rosemary
- ½ teaspoon of minced garlic
- 2 pounds of roast beef
- 1/3 cup of soy sauce

Directions:

1. Combine the soy sauce, bouillon, rosemary, and garlic together in a mixing bowl.
2. Turn on your instant pot. Place the roast and pour enough water to cover the roast; gently stir to mix well. Seal it tight.
3. Click the "MEAT/STEW" Cooking function; set the pressure level to "HIGH" and set the cooking time to 35 minutes. Let the pressure build to cook the ingredients. Once done, click the "CANCEL" setting and then click the "NPR" Cooking function to release the pressure naturally.
4. Gradually open the lid, and shred the meat. Mix in the shredded meat back in the potting mix and stir well. Transfer in serving containers. Serve warm.

Nutrition (for 100g):

- Calories 423
- Fat 14g
- Carbohydrates 12g
- Protein 21g
- Sodium 884mg

83. Rosemary Beef Chuck Roast

Preparation Time: 5 minutes
Cooking Time: 45 minutes
Servings: 5-6
Difficulty Level: Average
Ingredients:

- 3 pounds of chuck beef roast
- 3 garlic cloves
- ¼ cup balsamic vinegar
- 1 sprig of fresh rosemary
- 1 sprig of fresh thyme
- 1 cup of water
- 1 tablespoon of vegetable oil
- Salt and pepper to taste

Directions:

1. Chop slices in the beef roast and place the garlic cloves in them. Rub the roast with herbs, black pepper, and salt. Preheat your instant pot using the sauté setting and pour the oil. When warmed, mix in the beef roast and stir-cook until browned on all sides. Add the remaining ingredients; stir gently.
2. Seal tight and cook on high for 40 minutes using a manual setting. Allow the pressure to release naturally, about 10 minutes. Uncover and put the beef roast on the serving plates, slice, and serve.

Nutrition (for 100g):

- Calories 542
- Fat 11.2g
- Carbohydrates 8.7g
- Protein 55.2g
- Sodium 710mg

84. Pork Chops and Tomato Sauce

Preparation Time: 10 minutes
Cooking Time: 20 minutes
Servings: 4
Difficulty Level: Easy
Ingredients:
- 4 pork chops, boneless
- 1 tablespoon of soy sauce
- ¼ teaspoon of sesame oil
- 1 and ½ cups of tomato paste
- 1 yellow onion
- 8 mushrooms, sliced

Directions:

1. In a bowl, mix pork chops with soy sauce and sesame oil, toss and leave aside for 10 minutes. Set your instant pot on sauté

mode, add pork chops, and brown them for 5 minutes on each side. Stir in onion, and cook for 1-2 minutes more. Add tomato paste and mushrooms, toss, cover, and cook on high for 8-9 minutes. Divide everything between plates and serve. Enjoy!

Nutrition (for 100g):

- Calories 300
- Fat 7g
- Carbohydrates 18g
- Protein 4g
- Sodium 801mg

85. Chicken with Caper Sauce

Preparation Time: 10 minutes
Cooking Time: 18 minutes
Servings: 5
Difficulty Level: Difficult
Ingredients:
For Chicken:

- 2 eggs
- Salt and ground black pepper, as required
- 1 cup of dry breadcrumbs
- 2 tablespoons of olive oil
- 1½ pounds of skinless, boneless chicken breast halves, pounded into ¾inch thickness and cut into pieces

For Capers Sauce:

- 3 tablespoons of capers
- ½ cup of dry white wine
- 3 tablespoons of fresh lemon juice
- Salt and ground black pepper, as required
- 2 tablespoons of fresh parsley, chopped

Directions:

1. For the chicken: in a shallow dish, add the eggs, salt, and black pepper and beat until well combined. In another shallow dish, place breadcrumbs. Soak the chicken pieces in an egg mixture, then coat with the breadcrumbs evenly. Shake off the excess breadcrumbs.
2. Cook the oil over medium heat and cook the chicken pieces for about 5-7 minutes per side or until desired doneness. With a slotted spoon, situate the chicken pieces onto a paper towel-lined plate. With a piece of foil, cover the chicken pieces to keep them warm.
3. In the same skillet, incorporate all the sauce ingredients except parsley and cook for about 2-3 minutes, stirring continuously. Mix in the parsley and remove it from heat. Serve the chicken pieces with the topping of capers sauce.

Nutrition (for 100g):

1. Calories 352
2. Fat 13.5g
3. Carbohydrates 1.9g
4. Protein 1.2g
5. Sodium 741mg

86. Turkey Burgers with Mango Salsa

Preparation Time: 15 minutes
Cooking Time: 10 minutes
Servings: 6
Difficulty Level: Easy
Ingredients:
- 1½ pounds of ground turkey breast
- 1 teaspoon of sea salt, divided
- ¼ teaspoon of freshly ground black pepper
- 2 tablespoons of extra-virgin olive oil
- 2 mangos, peeled, pitted, and cubed
- ½ red onion, finely chopped

- Juice of 1 lime
- 1 garlic clove, minced
- ½ jalapeño pepper, seeded and finely minced
- 2 tablespoons of chopped fresh cilantro leaves

Directions:

1. Form the turkey breast into 4 patties and season with ½ teaspoon of sea salt and pepper. Cook the olive oil in a nonstick skillet until it shimmers. Add the turkey patties and cook for about 5 minutes per side until browned. While the patties cook, mix the mango, red onion, lime juice, garlic, jalapeño, cilantro, and remaining ½ teaspoon of sea salt in a small bowl. Spoon the salsa over the turkey patties and serve.

Nutrition (for 100g):

- Calories 384
- Fat 3g
- Carbohydrates 27g
- Protein 34g
- Sodium 692mg

87. Herb-Roasted Turkey Breast

Preparation Time: 15 minutes
Cooking Time: 1½ hours (plus 20 minutes to rest)
Servings: 6
Difficulty Level: Average
Ingredients:
- 2 tablespoons of extra-virgin olive oil
- 4 garlic cloves, minced
- Zest of 1 lemon
- 1 tablespoon of chopped fresh thyme leaves
- 1 tablespoon of chopped fresh rosemary leaves
- 2 tablespoons of chopped fresh Italian parsley leaves
- 1 teaspoon of ground mustard

- 1 teaspoon of sea salt
- ¼ teaspoon of freshly ground black pepper
- 1 (6-pound) bone-in, skin-on turkey breast
- 1 cup of dry white wine

Directions:

1. Preheat the oven to 325°F. Combine the olive oil, garlic, lemon zest, thyme, rosemary, parsley, mustard, sea salt, and pepper. Brush the herb mixture evenly over the turkey breast's surface, and loosen the skin and rub underneath as well. Situate the turkey breast in a roasting pan on a rack, skin-side up.
2. Pour the wine into the pan. Roast for 1 to 1½ hours until the turkey reaches an internal temperature of 165 ° F. Pull out from the oven and set separately for 20 minutes, tented with aluminum foil to keep it warm, before carving.

Nutrition (for 100g):

- Calories 392
- Fat 1g
- Carbohydrates 2g
- Protein 84g
- Sodium 741mg

88. Chicken Sausage and Peppers

Preparation Time: 10 minutes
Cooking Time: 20 minutes
Servings: 6
Difficulty Level: Average
Ingredients:

- 2 tablespoons of extra-virgin olive oil
- 6 Italian chicken sausage links
- 1 onion
- 1 red bell pepper
- 1 green bell pepper
- 3 garlic cloves, minced

- ½ cup of dry white wine
- ½ teaspoon of sea salt
- ¼ teaspoon of freshly ground black pepper
- Pinch red pepper flakes

Directions:

1. Cook the olive oil on a large skillet until it shimmers. Add the sausages and cook for 5 to 7 minutes, occasionally turning, until browned, and they reach an internal temperature of 165°F. With tongs, remove the sausage from the pan and set it aside on a platter, tented with aluminum foil to keep warm.
2. Return the skillet to heat and mix in the onion, red bell pepper, and green bell pepper. Cook and occasionally stir until the vegetables begin to brown. Put in the garlic and cook for 30 seconds, stirring constantly.
3. Stir in the wine, sea salt, pepper, and red pepper flakes. Pull out and fold in any browned bits from the bottom of the pan. Simmer for about 4 minutes more, stirring, until the liquid reduces by half. Spoon the peppers over the sausages and serve.

Nutrition (for 100g):

- Calories 173
- Fat 1g
- Carbohydrates 6g
- Protein 22g
- Sodium 582mg

89. Chicken Piccata

Preparation Time: 10 minutes
Cooking Time: 15 minutes
Servings: 6
Difficulty Level: Average
Ingredients:
- ½ cup of whole-wheat flour
- ½ teaspoon of sea salt

- 1/8 teaspoon of freshly ground black pepper
- 1½ pounds of chicken breasts, cut into 6 pieces
- 3 tablespoons of extra-virgin olive oil
- 1 cup of unsalted chicken broth
- ½ cup of dry white wine
- Juice of 1 lemon
- Zest of 1 lemon
- ¼ cup of capers drained and rinsed
- ¼ cup of chopped fresh parsley leaves

Directions:

1. In a shallow dish, whisk the flour, sea salt, and pepper. Scour the chicken in the flour and tap off any excess. Cook the olive oil until it shimmers.
2. Put the chicken and cook for about 4 minutes per side until browned. Pull out the chicken from the pan and set it aside, tented with aluminum foil to keep warm.
3. Situate the skillet back to the heat and stir in the broth, wine, lemon juice, lemon zest, and capers. Use the side of a spoon scoop and fold in any browned bits from the pan's bottom. Simmer until the liquid thickens. Take out the skillet from the heat and take the chicken back to the pan. Turn to coat. Stir in the parsley and serve.

Nutrition (for 100g):

- Calories 153
- Fat 2g
- Carbohydrates 9g
- Protein 8g
- Sodium 692mg

90. One-Pan Tuscan Chicken

Preparation Time: 10 minutes
Cooking Time: 25 minutes

Servings: 6
Difficulty Level: Difficult
Ingredients:

- ¼ cup of extra-virgin olive oil, divided
- 1-pound of boneless, skinless chicken breasts, cut into ¾-inch pieces
- 1 onion, chopped
- 1 red bell pepper, chopped
- 3 garlic cloves, minced
- ½ cup of dry white wine
- 1 (14-ounce) can of crushed tomatoes, undrained
- 1 (14-ounce) can of chopped tomatoes, drained
- 1 (14-ounce) can of white beans, drained
- 1 tablespoon of dried Italian seasoning
- ½ teaspoon of sea salt
- 1/8 teaspoon of freshly ground black pepper
- 1/8 teaspoon of red pepper flakes
- ¼ cup of chopped fresh basil leaves

Directions:

1. Cook 2 tablespoons of olive oil until it shimmers. Mix in the chicken and cook until browned. Remove the chicken from the skillet and set it aside on a platter, tented with aluminum foil to keep warm.
2. Situate the skillet back to the heat and heat up the remaining olive oil. Add the onion and red bell pepper. Cook and rarely stir until the vegetables are soft. Put the garlic and cook for 30 seconds, stirring constantly.
3. Stir in the wine, and use the spoon's side to scoop out any browned bits from the bottom of the pan. Cook for 1 minute, stirring.
4. Mix in the crushed and chopped tomatoes, white beans, Italian seasoning, sea salt, pepper, and red pepper flakes. Allow to simmer. Cook for 5 minutes, stirring occasionally.
5. Put the chicken back and any juices that have been collected into the skillet. Cook until the chicken is cook through. Take out from the heat and stir in the basil before serving.

Nutrition (for 100g):

- Calories 271
- Fat 8g
- Carbohydrates 29g
- Protein 14g
- Sodium 596mg

Chapter 5. Dessert Recipes

91. Hearty Cashew and Almond butter

Preparation Time: 5 minutes
Cooking Time: Nil
Servings: 1 and ½ cups
Ingredients:

- 1 cup of almonds, blanched
- 1/3 cup of cashew nuts
- 2 tablespoons of coconut oil
- Sunflower seeds as needed
- ½ teaspoon of cinnamon

Directions:

1. Pre-heat your oven to 350 ° F.
2. Bake almonds and cashews for 12 minutes.
3. Let them cool.
4. Transfer to the food processor and add the remaining ingredients.
5. Add oil and keep blending until smooth.
6. Serve and enjoy!

Nutrition:

- Calories: 205
- Fat: 19g
- Carbohydrates: g
- Protein: 2.8g
- Sodium 9%

92. The Refreshing Nutter

Preparation Time: 10 minutes
Cooking Time: 0 minutes
Servings: 1
Ingredients:

- 1 tablespoon of chia seeds
- 2 cups of water
- 1 ounce of Macadamia Nuts
- 1-2 packets of Stevia, optional
- 1-ounce of hazelnut

Directions:

1. Add all the listed ingredients to a blender.
2. Blend on high until smooth and creamy.
3. Enjoy your smoothie.

Nutrition:

- Calories: 452
- Fat: 43g
- Carbohydrates: 15g
- Protein: 9g
- Sodium 1%

93. Elegant Cranberry Muffins

Preparation Time: 10 minutes
Cooking Time: 20 minutes
Servings: 24 muffins
Ingredients:

- 2 cups of almond flour
- 2 teaspoons of baking soda

- ¼ cup of avocado oil
- 1 whole egg
- ¾ cup of almond milk
- ½ cup of Erythritol
- ½ cup apple sauce
- Zest of 1 orange
- 2 teaspoons of ground cinnamon
- 2 cup of fresh cranberries

Directions:

1. Pre-heat your oven to 350 ° F.
2. Line a muffin tin with paper muffin cups and keep them on the side.
3. Add flour, baking soda and keep it on the side.
4. Take another bowl and whisk the remaining ingredients and add flour, mix well.
5. Pour batter into prepared muffin tin and bake for 20 minutes.
6. Once done, let it cool for 10 minutes.
7. Serve and enjoy!

Nutrition:

- Calories: 354
- Total Carbs: 7g
- Fiber: 2g
- Protein: 2.3g
- Fat: 7g
- Sodium 77%

94. Apple and Almond Muffins

Preparation Time: 10 minutes
Cooking Time: 20 minutes
Servings: 6 muffins

Ingredients:

- 6 ounces of ground almonds
- 1 teaspoon of cinnamon
- ½ teaspoon of baking powder
- 1 pinch of sunflower seeds
- 1 whole egg
- 1 teaspoon of apple cider vinegar
- 2 tablespoons of Erythritol
- 1/3 cup of apple sauce

Directions:

1. Pre-heat your oven to 350 ° F.
2. Line muffin tin with paper muffin cups, and keep them on the side.
3. Mix in almonds, cinnamon, baking powder, sunflower seeds and keep it on the side.
4. Take another bowl and beat in eggs, apple cider vinegar, apple sauce, Erythritol.
5. Add the mix to dry ingredients and mix well until you have a smooth batter.
6. Pour batter into the tin and bake for 20 minutes.
7. Once done, let them cool.
8. Serve and enjoy!

Nutrition:

- Calories: 234
- Total Carbs: 10
- Fiber: 4g
- Protein: 13g
- Fat: 17g
- Sodium 47%

95. Stylish Chocolate Parfait

Preparation Time: 2 hours
Cooking Time: nil
Servings: 4

Ingredients:

- 2 tablespoons of cocoa powder
- 1 cup of almond milk
- 1 tablespoon of chia seeds
- ½ teaspoon of vanilla extract

Directions:

1. Take a bowl and add cocoa powder, almond milk, chia seeds, vanilla extract, and stir.
2. Transfer to dessert glass and place in your fridge for 2 hours.
3. Serve and enjoy!

Nutrition:

- Calories: 130
- Fat: 5g
- Carbohydrates: 7g
- Protein: 16g
- Sodium 4%

96. Supreme Matcha Bomb

Preparation Time: 100 minutes
Cooking Time: Nil
Servings: 10
Ingredients:

- 3/4 cup of hemp seeds
- ½ cup of coconut oil
- 2 tablespoons of coconut almond butter
- 1 teaspoon of Matcha powder
- 2 tablespoons of vanilla bean extract
- Liquid stevia

Directions:

1. Take your blender/food processor and add hemp seeds, coconut oil, Matcha, vanilla extract, and stevia.
2. Blend until you have a nice batter and divide into silicon molds.
3. Melt coconut almond butter and drizzle on top.
4. Let the cups chill and enjoy!

Nutrition:

- Calories: 200
- Fat: 20g
- Carbohydrates: 3g
- Protein: 5g
- Sodium 6%

97. Mesmerizing Avocado and Chocolate Pudding

Preparation Time: 30 minutes
Cooking Time: Nil
Servings: 2
Ingredients:

- 1 avocado, chunked
- 1 tablespoon of natural sweetener such as stevia
- 2 ounces of cream cheese, at room temp
- ¼ teaspoon of vanilla extract
- 4 tablespoons of cocoa powder, unsweetened

Directions:

1. Blend listed ingredients in a blender until smooth.
2. Divide the mix between dessert bowls, chill for 30 minutes.
3. Serve and enjoy!

Nutrition:

- Calories: 281
- Fat: 27g
- Carbohydrates: 12g
- Protein: 8g
- Sodium 18%

98. Hearty Pineapple Pudding

Preparation Time: 10 minutes
Cooking Time: 5 hours
Servings: 4
Ingredients:

- 1 teaspoon of baking powder
- 1 cup of coconut flour
- 3 tablespoons of stevia
- 3 tablespoons of avocado oil
- ½ cup of coconut milk
- ½ cup of pecans, chopped
- ½ cup of pineapple, chopped
- ½ cup of lemon zest, grated
- 1 cup of pineapple juice, natural

Directions:

1. Grease Slow Cooker with oil.
2. Take a bowl and mix in flour, stevia, baking powder, oil, milk, pecans, pineapple, lemon zest, pineapple juice, and stir well.
3. Pour the mix into the Slow Cooker.
4. Place lid and cook on LOW for 5 hours.
5. Divide between bowls and serve.
6. Enjoy!

Nutrition:

- Calories: 188
- Fat: 3g
- Carbohydrates: 14g
- Protein: 5g
- Sodium 5%

99. Healthy Berry Cobbler

Preparation Time: 10 minutes
Cooking Time: 2 hours 30 minutes
Servings: 8
Ingredients:

- 1 ¼ cups of almond flour
- 1 cup of coconut sugar
- 1 teaspoon of baking powder
- ½ teaspoon of cinnamon powder
- 1 whole egg
- ¼ cup of low-fat milk
- 2 tablespoons of olive oil
- 2 cups of raspberries
- 2 cups of blueberries

Directions:

1. Take a bowl and add almond flour, coconut sugar, baking powder, and cinnamon.
2. Stir well.
3. Take another bowl and add egg, milk, oil, raspberries, blueberries, and stir.
4. Combine both of the mixtures.
5. Grease your Slow Cooker.
6. Pour the combined mixture into your Slow Cooker and cook on HIGH for 2 hours 30 minutes.
7. Divide between serving bowls and enjoy!

Nutrition:

- Calories: 250
- Fat: 4g
- Carbohydrates: 30g
- Protein: 3g
- Sodium 1%

100.   Tasty Poached Apples

Preparation Time: 10 minutes
Cooking Time: 2 hours 30 minutes
Servings: 8
Ingredients:

- 6 apples, cored, peeled, and sliced
- 1 cup of apple juice, natural
- 1 cup of coconut sugar
- 1 tablespoon of cinnamon powder

Directions:

1. Grease Slow Cooker with cooking spray.
2. Add apples, sugar, juice, cinnamon to your Slow Cooker.
3. Stir gently.
4. Place lid and cook on HIGH for 4 hours.
5. Serve cold and enjoy!

Nutrition:

- Calories: 180
- Fat: 5g
- Carbohydrates: 8g
- Protein: 4g
- Sodium 2%

CPSIA information can be obtained
at www.ICGtesting.com
Printed in the USA
BVHW011442100621
609008BV00015B/1064

9 781802 551693